LIF

MW01601946

THE WARTIME JOURNALS
OF AN ANESTHESIOLOGIST

LIFE AS TRAUMA

THE WARTIME JOURNALS
OF AN ANESTHESIOLOGIST

by

Sarah Z. Mitić

TRANSLATED BY
Sarah Zorica Mitić
Simhe Levi Bogdanovich
Marija Stevanovich

EDITED BY
Milo Yelesiyevich

Unwritten History, Inc.
Chicago, Illinois

These journals were written during the time the events being described were taking place. The first part of the text was published in Serbia in 1997 under the title Iz Krajine koja više ne postoji (From Krajina, Which No Longer Exists) *by Filip Višnjić Publishers.*

In Norway, the entire text (Parts I, II and III) was published in 2008 under the title Mellom to tarer (Between Two Teardrops).

An abridged version was published in Denmark in 2009 under the title Tears.

Excerpts from the text were published in the periodical Duga (Rainbow) *in 1993 and 1994.*

Excerpts from the text were presented on the talk show Crni biseri (Black Pearls) *with Vanja Bulić in 1993, 1995, and 1997.*

Excerpts from the text were presented on Radio Politika: These Are the Nineties *(1993).*

Excerpts from the text were broadcast in the program On the Other Side of the Law *on Pančevo TV in 1994.*

Portions of the text were broadcast on Channel 5, TV Niš in 1996.

Photo Layout:
Every effort has been made by the publisher to trace the holder of the copyright for photographs numbered 7, 8, 9, 12, 13, 14, 15, 16, 25, and 26. As it stands now, the sources remain unknown. This omission will be rectified in future editions.

The Front Cover incorporates a photograph taken at the Exhibition *Odbrana 78* which was mounted by the Ministry of Defense of Serbia. The source for the Back Cover image is Deposit Photos.

Unwritten History, Inc.
P.O. Box 6753
Chicago, IL 60680-6753
unwrittenhistory@hotmail.com
website: www.unwrittenhistory.com

CONTENTS

Illustrations follow page 212.

FOREWORD

This powerful memoir by Sarah Mitić provides a firsthand account of the dreadful violence and bloodshed that followed the breakup of Yugoslavia. The author was a Serbian medical doctor who volunteered to serve on the battle fronts of the conflict. She kept a diary that forms the basis of this remarkable book. In addition to detailed accounts of the horrors of tending to the military and civilian casualties while under constant bombardment and the threat of being overrun by hostile forces, she proves to be an astute observer of the human condition during times of extreme psychological stress and physical terror.

However, perhaps the lasting value of this book will be that it is an eye-witness account of the cynicism and double standards practiced by our western political leaders and media in placing all of the responsibility of the conflict on the Serbian side. The betrayal and demonization of the Serbian people who had sacrificed so much in two world wars by supporting the western democracies were culminated by the massive ethnic cleansing of the Serbian people from their historic homeland in Croatia and the seventy-eight days and nights of the shameful and illegal bombing of the very people who had been their loyal allies

It is unlikely that there will ever be a truthful accounting of who was really responsible for the Balkan wars of the early 1990s, but Sarah Mitić's book may well be the beginning of a wider understanding of how and why NATO, in a desperate effort to justify its continuing existence, was prepared to cause such death and destruction to thousands of innocents on all sides of the conflict in order to support an outright fascist Croatian regime, and an extremist Muslim leader. Dr. Mitić's book is a personal experience but her story deserves a wide readership for the universal lessons she reveals within its pages.

James Bissett
Canadian Ambassador to Yugoslavia (1990–1992)

PART ONE

1. The Most Innocent Victims

I rush downstairs. The wailing ambulance siren is summoning us to the Emergency Room where medics are carrying in two tent flaps that hold the wounded. Blankets have been thrown over them. I sharply express my disapproval of covering the patients during transport. I abruptly fling back the canvas. A stabbing pain in my stomach doubles me over. I can't stand up straight. The girl's face is uninjured but her skull is open and her brains are oozing out. She has no torso because her smashed head has been rammed all the way down into her pelvis. I bite my lip so hard that it starts bleeding. I look at the other small mass of flesh and bones. The boy is alive. He's moving slightly and moaning. They are a brother and sister who were playing in the mountains where they stumbled upon an unexploded bomb.

All that was left of them after the explosion was blood and flesh mingled with dust. They gathered what remained of these children in two tent flaps and brought them to the hospital. The girl is going to the morgue; the boy has to be operated on.

We treat the boy's wounds mechanically and take him to the Operating Room. The upshot of our hard work — which lasted for several hours — is the amputation of his legs above the knee; his right arm up to the elbow; and even though both his eyes have been injured, there's a chance that one might be saved. He's bandaged up like a mummy, lying in bed under an oxygen tent. He is six years old.

I'm standing at his bedside, still biting my lip, but my hands are trembling now. I'm a doctor but I can't take this. I'd give up everything for the chance to make sure no one in the world ever has to experience this again. I fight back the tears, but they come running down my nose anyway. I'm sniffling audibly.

The boy hears me and he moans quietly.

"Why are you crying, Mom? I can feel wind blowing on my nose. Why can't I see you? Touch me.... Where's sis?"

"Go to sleep, my child." I say. "Your eyes are bandaged, that's why you can't see anything. Your little sister is at home... Now go to sleep, my little one."

I reach out and touch his neck because that's the only unbandaged spot on his body.

"Mom, why don't you kiss me?" he asks.

I can't bear it any longer. I clasp my hands tightly and move away from the bed. An attending nurse puts her arms around me. She leads me, my head hanging down, to a room where I can recover. I can't see anything.... I seek refuge in the toilet. That's where I start screaming:

"O, my God!? I've had enough. I can't take it anymore! Why children?"

I squat down on the floor beside the toilet and I cry … and I cry … and I cry. When I finally get up, I'm speechless. My throat hurts, my face is flushed crimson, and my eyelids are swollen. I just can't calm down. I run to my room. I lie down on the bed fully dressed, cover myself with a blanket, curl up, and then fall half asleep. I can't even move until the evening. I'm unable to work. I've gone to pieces.

* * * *

When I set out on this journey, some acquaintances asked me: *You're probably expecting to come back home with medals, aren't you? You're going to be the glamorous new SUBNOR.*[1] I wouldn't have told this story to such people. They wouldn't have understood it, anyway. If any of their children had been killed, would they then still be preoccupied with their own selfish interests?! That's when I catch myself: *what am I thinking?* How cruel and embittered I have become. God, please don't allow me to judge people who think differently or else I'm going to turn into malevolent creature that goes around in rage and despair and slashes and stabs random passers-by with a sword! What are the concerns of my acquaintances in Serbia? What are my concerns? Why is everything so complicated? Why are so many questions running through my head? It hurts so much that I feel like screaming. It hurts because my friends in Serbia think I have a thirst for adventure. They haven't grasped the gravity of the situation: the people in Krajina are fighting for their lives and they need help desperately.

One of my distant cousins is ten years old. She mistook a similar bomb for a toy, which severed her right hand. The doctors in Belgrade barely managed to save her left hand.

War teaches us harsh realities: our existence is transitory; life is easy to lose; death, chaos, and despair rule. It's difficult to explain this to uninformed outsiders. The war hasn't touched their lives. News reports in the Serbian media distort the truth. My friends in Serbia perceive this war as something inconceivable that is taking place far, far away. In other words, the war doesn't really exist.

---

1. SUBNOR (*Savez udruženja boraca Narodnooslobodilačkog rata*) The League of WWII Veterans' Association.

They can't share the unendurable pain that threatens to paralyze me and perhaps, in the long run, threatens to defeat me.

These innocent children mistook bombs for toys. And I'm supposed to get a medal for this?! O lost and miserable generation!

The boy was transported to Belgrade. I can only imagine what fate held in store for him.

A doctor from the hospital calls me into his office for a *tête-à-tête*. He places a glass of hard liquor before me.

"Sit down. Have a drink!"

"Thank you," I reply apologetically. "I don't drink."

"Drink up and relax. We've all gone through this phase. You go through tough times. The pain makes you feel tense, and then you lose control. People vent or shout at co-workers. Some just cry, others break down, and still others go crazy," he tells me while holding my hands which are trembling uncontrollably. "Every emotional reaction is good. What comes afterward is much worse. You sink into indifference. You get used to death. Losing becomes routine. That's the greatest horror," he says after a pause. "I don't cry anymore."

He goes on: "You don't believe me? I used to cry, too. Tears don't solve anything. We can't overcome tragedy with tears. I never drank before. Now I drink! It makes me feel better, it warms me up. My eyes get misty but at least I can carry on.

"You volunteers come and go, but I have to stay here," he continues. "I have to stay healthy, normal, and ready to help. You see only blood, maiming, and death. I see all that *plus* the deaths of relatives, neighbors, and friends. I was born here. I live here. This is my home."

I'm ashamed. I should be the one comforting him, but he's comforting me, instead!

He's a young man. He's hunched over, staring into the void.

* * * *

It's a cold winter night. We had worked from morning until late into the night. I went from one OR to another. I was dead on my feet. We ventilated patients by hand in order to save oxygen. I rest my head on a pillow for just a moment, and I keep ventilating the patient with my eyes closed. Overcome with exhaustion, I suddenly drift off. Then I see the patient with his head hanging over the bed, his face completely blue. His eyes are wide open. He almost falls over on me. *O, my God!* I think. I've killed him! I'm afraid to look and see if the patient is already dead. Why didn't the surgeons see it coming? When I look around fearfully, the patient isn't there. I'm not in the OR any more. An anesthetist orderly carried me out of the OR and laid me down in the corridor to sleep. He's now working in my stead. I've been dreaming.

Even though I'm at the end of my tether, I make an effort to get up off the floor and peek into the OR to make sure that everything is all right. I'm happy when I see that wonderful military orderly who relieved me ventilating the patient. He waves his hand, signaling that it was okay for me to rest a little longer. I'm so grateful to him.

I've been working for more than two weeks without a break, with perhaps only two or three hours of sleep a night. I'm in good shape because I was once an athlete but I've finally reached the limits of my physical endurance. Rest has become vitally important. I start to shiver uncontrollably. I cover myself with a non-sterile compress and curl up on a field bed. I'm running a fever. I can't take any more.

Then the telephone starts ringing. I barely manage to get up.

"Is this the Intensive Care Unit?" asks the switchboard operator.

"Yes!"

"You have a long-distance call from Canada. Hold the line, please."

I hear a loud noise on the receiver, then a voice:

"May I speak to Dr. Sarah Z. Mitić from Smederevo?"

"This is Sarah speaking. How may I help you?"

My heart leaps with joy as I recognize his voice: "Is that you?"

"Yes!" answers my uncle, who emigrated to Canada years ago.

"I have to tell you that I'm proud of you," he says through his sobs. "I wish I were there. I was born there. My father was killed there. Thank you for being there."

My uncle, as many of my other family members, had to leave the country because he held opinions that differed from the ones held by those in power. My grandfather was a soldier here. He was also killed here. And now I'm fighting in a new war in the same place. History *does* repeat itself.

We're unable to continue our conversation because we're both crying. Pain and joy mingle and resound against the doors and windows. The beating of my heart fills the room. How did he find me?

This one telephone call reinvigorates me and gets me back on my feet. I don't know where this energy comes from but it comes in wave after wave of warmth.

I go back to the OR and relieve the anesthetist.

The War Starts while I'm on Vacation

We were vacationing in Greece in the summer of 1991 when news of the turmoil back home reached us. My husband Miroslav and I were with our two small daughters on the island of Tassos, where we were relaxing, walking along the beach, and sunbathing. Miroslav went to buy his daily batch of newspapers. His Serbo-Chilean temperament, his demanding job as Director of the Public Revenue Office in Smederevo, his added responsibilities of acting Deputy Director of the Revenue Office of Serbia, as well as his being a member of the local municipal government kept Miroslav high-strung. But I didn't expect to hear him scream:

WAR IN YUGOSLAVIA!

The news struck terror into our hearts. Common sense invited us to deny these reports. Miroslav, whom we all called "Cile,"[2] had long ago predicted the disintegration of Yugoslavia. Now foreign newspapers were publishing this as a news item, so his prediction was coming to pass. He was paralyzed, dazed by disbelief and bewilderment. Tears were streaking his handsome face. I was shaken, too, but I embraced him and caressed him and tried to calm him down. A growing sense of powerlessness began suffocating me. I was terrified! The children were frightened, and they were staring at us with unconcealed confusion. My youngest child placed her small hand into mine. In one fell moment, we lost the most basic sense of security, which we once took for granted.

I wanted to return to Yugoslavia immediately. Cile agreed at first, but then his protective spirit prevailed. He insisted that I remain with the children in Greece while he returned to Serbia alone. He planned to sell everything we owned and then return to join us. He wanted the children far away from the chaos that is sure to follow. History has shown many a time that a small fire in the Balkans can quickly flare up into a dangerous conflagration.

"And what if you don't return?" I asked anxiously.

"You'll stay here and manage somehow. What's important is that you and the children are far away from the war!"

I didn't think this was an acceptable option. A wife doesn't leave her husband in times of difficulty, and a doctor doesn't leave patients just because a war is going on. No, I'm not going

---

2. Cile, pronounced *Tseelay*.

to be sheltered from this war. If my fate is to be killed, then I'll die with my fellow countrymen. I'm worried about our children, of course. They have no choice in this matter.

"What 'people' are you talking about, Sarah?" Cile asked me ironically when I spoke to him of my feelings. "You know very well how arrogantly those officials treated you!"

Cile was referring to a series of humiliations to which I had been subjected by Serbian authorities when I had to compete for a place in the regular allotment of apartments for medical personnel. I was an anesthesiologist, an indispensable part of the surgical team at the hospital where I was working, and I was also next on the apartment list. But corruption is rampant, which effectively knocked me off the top of the list. I have no political pull. My only advantage was professional expertise. After I lost my spot, I found myself on the street with two children in the middle of winter. That was how I met Cile. He rescued me from further humiliations as well as from the cold. I don't dare even think of what could have happened to me and the children if he hadn't helped us.

Now my husband was extremely upset.

"Milošević is a foreign mercenary. He's a traitor to the Serbian people! Haven't you seen the Constitution he rammed down our throat? It's Communist nonsense! *Serbia is a country of all its citizens.* No! *Serbia is a state composed of Serbs and all other nationalities!* That's what a *real* patriot would have written!" Miroslav raged.

Miroslav continued venting. He was actually shouting. On the one hand, I never thought that there was anything suspicious about the new Constitution; on the other hand, however, I don't know much about the law. I really didn't know what to say.

We hurried back to the hotel, hastily paid our bill, and then began our journey back home to Smederevo, which was once the medieval capital of Serbia. It was also where Miroslav was born. I was born and raised nearby in Belgrade, the Yugoslav capital, but now I'm working in Smederevo as an anesthesiologist at the Clinical Center at the Serbian Teaching Hospital.

As soon as we crossed the Macedonian-Serbian border, Cile stopped our silver-grey Toyota Corolla and the four of us got out of the car in solemn silence, knelt, and kissed the ground. Back on Serbian soil at last!

Cile fervently crossed himself and prayed for the salvation of Yugoslavia, especially Serbia. I thought he had seen too many patriotic war movies. To me, he appeared histrionic. Miroslav has a gift for drama. His mind overemphasizes, sharpens, and distills, and then he adds drama to an already grave situation. I chose to remain silent.

I'm in absolute denial. I'm unwilling to believe that war can break out in Yugoslavia. I grew up wearing a red scarf.[3] I learned *brotherhood and unity*[4] here in my native Serbia, where it was transmitted by edifying stories. When I was in high school I learned by heart a long poem called *The Pit*[5] which was written to memorialize the fascist Ustaše[6] crimes against Serbs in Croatia during World War II. I went on school excursions to Kragujevac to honor the memory of the 4,000 students who were executed there by Germans soldiers. We visited Jasenovac, where the Croatians killed 700,000 Serbs, Jews, and Roma. Ever since I was a child, I was taught to believe in the unity of Yugoslavia's peoples.

---

3. *red scarf*, emblem of the Pioneers, the Communist youth organization similar to the Boy and Girl Scouts.
4. *brotherhood and unity*, the official Communist slogan for the post-WWII policy of quelling animosity between ethnic groups in the former Yugoslavia.
5. *The Pit* (Jama), a poem by Ivan Goran Kovačić.
6. *Ustaše*, Fascist Croats who were allied to the Nazis during WWII.

Marshal Tito united us under a unified Yugoslav national identity. I was a good student, so I was singled out for additional training in political orientation camps in Tito's hometown of Kumrovec. I can't tell you how many times I've run the Yugoslav flag up a flagpole at these camps after we had gotten up at daybreak for work details. At first, I participated with a pickaxe in my hand; then as a student with a pen; and later as doctor with a syringe. I helped build this country and I worked hard for it.

I was proud that Marshal Tito, along with Jawaharlal Nehru, Sukarno, and Nasser, founded the Non-Aligned Movement (NAM) in 1961 in Belgrade — my home town. Ultimately, 120 countries, or 55% of the world's population, joined the NAM which provided a sense of security and strength in unity to smaller, militarily weaker nations. It represented a balance of power that checked imperialism and colonialism. We members of the post-war generation are still proud this. It's unthinkable that any of the Yugoslav peoples would actually want to replace Yugoslavia with smaller, weaker states. It's beyond my comprehension that people could even consider destroying all that we had been taught to cherish. Serbia has a long tradition of independence, but *unity* is the backbone of Yugoslavia.

On the way home, I kept telling myself that things were going to settle down, and that once we arrived in Smederevo, we were going to hear that this brouhaha was just a flash in the pan.

But in Serbia, we found out what we were unable to learn from foreign newspaper accounts. The Territorial Defense Forces (TO)[7] are a separate division of the Armed Forces of the Socialist Federal Republic of Yugoslavia. These forces act as a Home Guard, and they roughly correspond to an official gov-

---

7. *TO*, i.e., an acronym for *Teritorialna odbrana*.

ernmental paramilitary force. TOs had been established in each of Yugoslavia's constituent republics. The regular army of the Federation is the Yugoslav People's Army (JNA), which also maintains its own reserve forces. What happened was the TO of Slovenia launched an attack against the JNA barracks where young recruits who were doing their regular military service were stationed. The JNA retreated from Slovenia, but the renegade Slovenian TO Forces pressed on with their attacks. At the Holmec border crossing with Austria, the Slovenian TO killed JNA soldiers who had surrendered with white flags in their hands. Similar killings of JNA soldiers were taking place at many other border crossing posts along the Austrian frontier.

I can't comprehend this. If the JNA is withdrawing, why are the Slovenians still killing JNA soldiers? It's monstrous! And why is this taking place in Slovenia, which has always been the wealthiest region in Yugoslavia? What do they want so badly that they need to go to such extremes? Despite my growing sense of disbelief and denial, I keep asking questions that no one is able to answer. I still love Slovenia.

The JNA is mobilizing troops in Serbia. They are recruiting volunteers to join the regular army to defend Yugoslavia from separatists in the other republics, especially Croatia. Soon, television news and newspapers articles report that Croatian hooligans killed a JNA soldier in May 1991. They strangled, with their bare hands, a young Macedonian soldier during a regularly scheduled military parade. Hooligans jumped on a tank, dragged out a young soldier in front of an enraged crowd, and strangled him. Bystanders applauded the murder. Is this the way to achieve independence?

Even though the video footage clearly showed the faces of these brazen murderers, no one in Serbia had seen it. I can't understand why this story is finally being reported now after so much time has passed. Why didn't we hear about it when it happened? Had the engineering of public opinion begun that long ago? How can we possibly know what information isn't reaching us? And what stories are we being told that are completely fictional? Yugoslavia is coming apart at the seams.

2. My First Trip to Krajina

The Serbian Krajina is largely composed of mountainous terrain between northern Croatia and the Adriatic coast. Its southern boundary skirts the Bosnian border. In the sixteenth century, the Austro-Hungarian Empire encouraged Serbs to settle this border region which was administered by the military. Here, Serbs acted as a bulwark against Ottoman Turkish incursions. After World War I, Krajina, as part of the former Austro-Hungarian Empire, joined the Kingdom of Serbs, Croats, and Slovenes, which later became the Socialist Republic of Yugoslavia. Croatia now wants independence. Nevertheless, history doesn't help me, a Yugoslav who believes in brotherhood and unity, understand why these killings have begun.

Killing and fairness are utterly incompatible. When hatred and killing start, value systems are destroyed. Truth dies as soon as war starts, just as it has throughout history. Whenever there are no answers, everyone is to blame. To me, journalists on all sides are among the first killers in this war because they present a distorted picture of reality. Lies are journalism's most insidious weapon.

Health officials began using all media to make daily public service announcements calling on anesthesiologists and surgeons to volunteer in hospitals in Croatia and Bosnia & Herzegovina, where they were desperately needed. The number of wounded soldiers and injured civilian victims keeps growing but there are not enough doctors to provide emergency medical treatment. I attempted, as if I were in a trance and guided by unbearable anguish, several times to set out on organized expeditions to the scene of the conflict in Krajina. Yes, I have small children but I also have to think about the many other children, as well, who don't have anyone to help them. My children are provided for and safe. I'm a doctor, I tell myself: I must participate on the right side — on the side of humanity.

I'm still working at the Clinical Center. I also keep up with news about emerging events in Krajina. People around me are not as interested in what's going on as I am. I'm more upset than the others because I have family there. My mother was born in Krajina, so perhaps that's the reason it's so dear to me. But my colleagues' indifference hurts.

Miroslav is also upset. He has publicly said that Milošević is a traitor to the Serbian people and that he has let the people of Krajina down.

"A real leader who cares about his people would have mobilized the population, put everyone in uniform, given them arms and said: *Okay, if you want to fight, here we are. Instead of attacking Serbian women and children in Krajina, come and fight us!* And what does that weasel do? He calls for volunteers! What can a handful of volunteers do against the professional Croatian Army?"

Miroslav rages continually against the government's policies. I'm afraid that this might lead to tragic consequences for him as well as perhaps for me. People around him seem to agree with everything he's saying, but behind his back it's probably a different story.

The Serbs in Serbia are not willing to go to Krajina to fight for their fellow Serbs. I'm ashamed of these people. I'm ashamed of myself, too. Miroslav is not the father of my two children, so my small family could be imperiled if I were to go to Krajina. I can't even talk to Miroslav about my dilemma. Although he rails about Milošević's betrayal, I'm not sure how he would react if I were to tell him that I had to leave now. He's going to lose the most sympathetic audience he ever had.

I try to lead a normal life, but every now and then I hear a news item on TV or I speak with a refugee from Krajina who tells me incredible stories. It just breaks my heart all over again. At the hairdresser's, a woman was talking about Krajina. The Croats are persecuting Serbs: they're firing them from jobs; arresting them arbitrarily; and refusing them medical treatment. That's why this woman had to come to Serbia in the first place — for kidney dialysis. As I listened to her, I felt more strongly than ever that it was my duty to do something. I'm ashamed of my procrastination.

The situation is now clear. I have to help the people in Krajina.

I feel stronger and more composed after making the decision to go. Now I have to make practical arrangements for my trip and I have to plan things in the best possible way for my family to cope with my absence.

How are my children going to react? I embrace them, and I feel my eyes filling with tears at the very thought of leaving them. I begin to wonder whether the poems and tales of Serbian valor are just cherished fictions. They are not. No one ever gladly went to war. Courageous individuals join the struggle, but most people remain indifferent until war touches them personally. Perhaps I can set an example. My ancestors were brave. Can I be brave, too?

My first questions are: *How am I going to get there? Whom should I contact?* The answers came of their own accord. I ran into a doctor from the Military Hospital in Belgrade where I used to work. He told me that a group of volunteer doctors had already left for Knin. I immediately understand that I can join them. These are people I know and it will be easy to work with them. I think I'll be safe with them, too.

My children are already asleep when I sit on the floor beside the telephone. Knin, at the center of fighting in Krajina, is 800 kilometers away. I'm prepared to spend hours trying to place the call, but the telephone rings immediately and I get a connection right away. I ask to speak to Dr. Tomanović, the doctor on duty in the Anesthesia Department. By sheer chance, he's a doctor whom I already know and like. He advises me of his situation. His wife is going to have a baby, but neither he nor his wife has relatives who can help. He has to go back home, but he hasn't found a replacement yet.

"I'll replace you," I say without hesitation.

Dr. Tomanović is delighted. He knows that I'm going to rise to the challenge. He's not even surprised by my call, he says, because I have a reputation as a person who's willing to help. We immediately work out the details. After I hang up, I feel a friendly current running through the darkness from Smederevo all the way to Knin.

I quickly draw up a plan. First, I have to get a leave of absence from the hospital; then I have to find someone to look after my children; and lastly, I have to figure out how I'm going to cover my travel expenses. Of course, I also have to see how Cile is going to react. He might try to stop me from going. My children may cry. What if I can't bear leaving them? Even so, my inner voice is stronger than the actual obstacles I face.

I didn't sleep much that night. In the morning, I tell Miroslav about my decision. He embraces me.

"I'm proud of you," he says with tears welling his eyes. "It'll be hard for us without you, but I won't stop you from going. But who's going to take care of the children? You know that I'm not much help there," he says, grinning sheepishly.

That day, I also spoke to my family about it. My mother and brother disapproved, while my father — who's a disabled WWII veteran — says that he'll look after Ljuba, my younger daughter, who's only four years old. My father knows that nothing can stop me once I make up my mind.

My eldest daughter Marija is ten. She's going to school in Smederevo. She'll stay in our apartment with Cile. The woman who looks after my daughters while I'm at work agreed to take care of her, so that part worked out easily.

Miroslav's family, however, ridiculed me. At one family gathering, his brother said sarcastically to me:

"Ha, you're going to Krajina to pick up a couple of medals so that you can brag about it later. No one is going to be able to put up with you then!"

Miroslav didn't have a good relationship with his brother. He took the remark as a deliberate provocation. So, Miroslav became upset and insisted on leaving. But before we left, I gave his family a taste of my own indignation:

"If you're so envious about the possibility of my receiving a medal, then why don't you come along and get one yourself?"

We left, but we could hear the guests speaking among themselves: "She's a damn fool! All she's going to do is enflame ethnic tensions."

Tears were streaming down my face. Miroslav, one step ahead of me, angrily muttered: "Idiots! It didn't even occur to them that you could get killed, that I could lose the woman I love...."

He addressed me tenderly: "Just promise me that you won't expose yourself unnecessarily to danger. Remember, you're going to serve as a doctor. You're not a soldier; you're a doctor."

My Director, whose family hails from Krajina, gave my request for a leave of absence an even chillier response. He simply refused to grant it, and he refused to take the matter up with the Ministry of Health. The smooth operation of his department in the Clinical Center in Serbia was by far more important to him than the needs of the people in Krajina. He said that the government ought to take care of those people, and he mocked my decision to volunteer to go to a war zone. It was ridiculous, he said, for me to request a leave of absence so that I could go off on an "adventure."

I'm furious and heartbroken. Professor Cvetković, the Director of the Ophthalmology Department, also heard about the argument I had with my boss. He stepped in to help me. I worked with him for several years, often in complete secrecy outside of normal office hours for reasons of patient confidentiality when political figures and their families were concerned. The Professor's trust in me, a young doctor, was naturally a great honor and it increased my self-confidence. At that time, Professor Cvetković was President of the Serbian Parliament. He was calling for the first ever democratic parliamentary elections in Serbia.

Although Professor Cvetković remained silent during the meeting with the Director, he later asked to speak with me privately in his office. He quizzed me about my decision to go to the front. He wanted to know with whom I was going. I had no secrets: I simply held the conviction that I was supposed to help wherever help was needed. I was going there on my own. I planned buy my own bus ticket to Knin, where I was going to replace a doctor who was returning to Belgrade. I planned to live in the hospital. What the department director had said was not as important as what Professor Cvetković said.

"I wouldn't help you if I thought you were going with bandits or criminals from Arkan's Tigers or the White Eagles," said Professor Cvetković gravely.

The Tigers are a well-run paramilitary organization led by Želkjo Ražnjatović, AKA Arkan, a known criminal who had lived in Sweden and elsewhere in Europe. In Yugoslavia, he was rumored to have taken care of dirty work for the authorities. He was born in Montenegro, but had settled in Belgrade where he ran several night-clubs. A few well-known athletes allied themselves with Arkan after he began touting himself as a great patriot and protector of Serbs under attack in other Yugoslav republics. Since the recruitment drive had failed in Serbia, criminals and other shady groups began filling the ranks, instead.

The White Eagles are patriotic volunteers led by Vojislav Šešelj, an attorney. Born in Bosnia and Herzegovina, he received his Doctorate in Law at the age of twenty-five, which made him the youngest candidate ever to receive a Ph.D. in Yugoslavia. He's brilliant, but he was traumatized by vicious attacks during his youth. He was raped and tortured in prison at the hands of Bosnian Muslims. Since it was forbidden in Tito's Yugoslavia to comment negatively about non-Serbs, the perpetrators of these crimes were never punished. At the start of the war, Šešelj formed his own volunteer army that took the name White Eagles. They are far from professional, and they cannot at all be considered a crack military unit. Their hallmark is their patriotism and their desire to protect Serbs under attack from other nationalities. Many other such factions appeared. To join any of them is unthinkable.

"But, of course," said Professor Cvetković. "I wasn't expecting you to go with them."

He smiled, then quickly became serious again.

"And don't even think of having your picture taken with anyone in the Army. No one knows who's going to come out on the winning side," he said thoughtfully. "God help you … don't get yourself killed over there. You really have to be careful. Make sure that no pictures of you with anyone involved in this war ever surface. There's always a chance that you or your children could be brought to trial because of it."

He paused to let that sink in. Then he continued:

"Beware. Photographs are historical documents and they don't explain the attendant circumstances. They can, instead, be presented as irrefutable facts."

He rose to his feet.

"I'll take you to the Ministry of Health, and I will personally request that they send you there officially from Serbia, so you're not just a volunteer, even though that's what you really are. If you go officially, you'll have better protection under the law. You'll get travel orders and you'll continue to receive your salary during your absence. Otherwise, you'll go bankrupt."

I would not have been able to go without his intervention.

I soon received from the Ministry of Health my official travel orders, which enabled my children to inherit my pension if I were to be killed. Had I left without these orders, my children would have lost that right and they would have been left without financial resources.

"If I were killed...." For the first time, I face the fact that I may be wounded or die there. It all sounds distant and unreal. I'm still motivated and ready to go. I'm not afraid. I won't allow myself to consider the possibility of being killed. I focus instead on my mission.

I managed to finalize all the preparations, so I was ready to leave in October. First, a heart-breaking farewell to my children and Cile at the Belgrade bus terminal. Then, I boarded a bus whose door was barely working. This was how my journey to Knin began. My decision triggered an avalanche of gossip and disapproval. Does the word "patriotism" mean anything to these people?

I'm leaving Serbia behind.

3. Journey to Knin

The ramshackle bus we're riding reminds me of the one used in the film *Who's That Singing over There?* (*Ko To Tamo Peva?*). I have a stomach ache. I feel as if I had ingested stones. I'm frightened when the bus crosses the border into Bosnia. There's no turning back now. We pass Muslim, Croatian, and Serbian guard posts and check points. All of them search us.

We're going along a narrow road where we encounter a column of chilblained and bewildered refugees.

I see them through the misty windows of the bus as if it were a dream. They're taking small, anguished, reluctant steps forward. They've been forced to leave. I can't believe this is happening. My traveling companions become tearful as they watch a passing column of tractors pulling open trailers, where old men are sitting on top or lying down bundled in sheepskin overcoats and blankets. Children are peeping out from underneath warm blankets like mice. I can see the misty clouds of their breath. It's cold. Winter is drawing near

The refugees' miserable belongings are piled on a somber procession of tractors: bundles of clothing, footwear, and white pressure cookers are easily be distinguished. The women have wrinkled faces that seem to have grown old overnight; they have dull, absent expressions, and they are staring blankly into the distance because they have left their souls behind in the homes they abandoned. They are traveling into the unknown, leaving the places where they were born, where they married, where they gave birth to their children. They wouldn't have had time to feed or water their livestock; their houses have been left open. Their homes don't belong to them anymore. Someone turned a leaf in the Doomsday Book, which resulted in their lives being hurled into a dark abyss. Are their Croatian neighbors going to take care of those homes until the war is over? The column of people stretches into a long undulating line over the countryside.

"God willing, we'll endure! Just let our children live ... let them live!" says one woman, whose prayer vanishes into the frozen earth.

"Bastards!" a passenger mutters in a tone of anger and resignation. "Where are all these poor people going to go now!?"

The other passengers are angry too. Helplessness and pain arouse anger as well as the urge to avenge such humiliating treatment.

The sky is grey. Now and then, telltale raindrops streak the dusty windows of the bus.

We drive down narrow dirt roads and over bridges where cars are allowed to pass only one at a time. And whenever the bus crosses such a bridge, the planks groan beneath its weight. Any one of those bridges could have collapsed at any given moment, but none did. Two good-natured drivers from Donji Lapac are driving the bus in shifts. They're reliable, careful, and prudent. They're going to bring us to our destination. By preserving their own lives they're going to preserve ours, as well.

We skirt all of the larger towns. It's dangerous because ethnic tensions are running high and violence is likely. In these circumstances, the population is being forced to differentiate itself ethnically. The tension has increased to the point where shootings are taking place. But we can't avoid passing through Tuzla. It's ominously quiet. The wind is threatening to raise a dust storm. Traffic signs have been removed. It's a silent, featureless town where the rare passerby hurries along, focusing exclusively on his destination. I think of a college friend who lives here. She's a Muslim. We got along well. We were good friends, in fact. I wonder: where is she now? Does she also think that I hate her because I'm Serb? I can't accept this. She's a kindred spirit. No media propaganda can take away our memories. Why would she hate me now?

* * * *

I'm suspicious of each and every one of the people on this bus. I can't figure out who they are or why they're traveling to a war zone. I keep to myself. I'm afraid of making a wrong move and triggering a detonator in someone's head. It could cost me my life. My own head is also full of prejudices about those who are starting war. It would be dumb to get myself killed on my way to Krajina before I even have a chance to fulfill my responsibilities. I'm afraid of the armed guards at check-points — because no one controls them.

The journey drags on. Late in the night, we come to a checkpoint manned by Serbian guards. We're in Serbian Krajina. The road is steep and winding. The hill above us is on fire. The bus driver explains:

"The Croats are launching flares from helicopters to start forest fires. Their saboteurs are infiltrating Serbian territory."

This is a clear signal that Serbs aren't safe in Croatia.

Long after midnight, we arrive in Knin. The bus stops at a bend in the road. The driver exits the bus with me and leads me to a small elevation, where he points out an illuminated building about a kilometer away.

"That's the new hospital," he says. "Over there, on the outskirts of town."

St. Sava Hospital

From a distance, the hospital reminds me of the VMA[8] in Belgrade. I wonder why there are so many lights on. Aren't they afraid of being bombed?

I'm carrying two bags: one has clothing and books, like M. Scott Peck's *The Road Less Traveled*, which I take everywhere; the other has medical supplies and medicine I'm donating to the hospital. I'm walking down the middle of an empty road. I'm afraid to use the sidewalk because there may be someone lurking in the shadows. I'm afraid to be walking alone in the dark but I forge ahead anyway. I keep looking straight ahead.

---

8.   VMA (*Vojna medicinksa akademija*), the Military Medical Academy.

The guard at the hospital entrance gives my identity documents a cursory glance. Then I enter the clean and spacious halls of St. Sava Hospital. A nurse leads me to the room where I'm going to be staying. My one friend here has left by helicopter to accompany wounded soldiers to Belgrade. I don't know anyone else. The room has a clean double bed with a bathroom and telephone — but there's no hot water. I get this room because I'm the only woman on the medical team. The doctor who was occupying it gallantly volunteered to move to a less desirable attic room.

I take a cold bath. A little later I go to the OR to have a look-see. I find out from the nurses that they have hot water. By morning, I'm part of the team.

The hospital is imposing. There are three nice, large operating rooms designed to meet international standards, as well as two smaller ones in the Emergency Room on the ground floor. When a patient is admitted, he is immediately taken to the ER, where all the other outpatient departments are located. There are sufficient amounts of medicine and supplies. Every morning, a staff meeting is held. The Director receives reports on admissions as well as the events that took place during the previous twenty-four hours, so a working plan is presented. Professional problems are resolved in a team context. This maintains order and discipline, but I'm surprised that they're able to stick to these procedures during wartime.

Apart from the hospital staff — I'm talking about people who didn't flee to Serbia or Croatia or even abroad — there's a team of doctors who came from the VMA. They've been working non-stop ever since ever since they arrived the beginning of the month. They're tired and depressed, but they don't speak of it. I fit into the team because I have nowhere else to go — I don't want to leave the safety of the hospital — I work day and night.

* * * *

I try my best to relieve the local doctors. Dr. Savo J., the Head of the Anesthesiology Department, is a peer. Dr. Savo and I are the same age, and we have the same number of years of professional service, yet we are both somehow still inexperienced. I was working in a large clinic with a far greater number of patients, while he was working here in a small town which had a population of less than ten thousand people. In any case, he's at home here. He's been working under these conditions for several months, which have toughened him up. I never leave his side if I can help it.

He has an inextinguishably positive attitude. We establish a cordial working relationship. He's very capable, and he's one of the best anesthesiologists that I've met in my short time here. Yet I find it strange that he's the Department Head. None of his positive character traits would have been considered as qualities meriting promotion in the politically charged atmosphere I had experienced in Belgrade.

Dr. Dragan P., the Hospital Director, has just been promoted from Department Head, which explains how Dr. Savo J. ended up as Head of Anesthesiology. Things haven't been easy for either of them. The political structures in Krajina are deteriorating. We're isolated — stranded on an island during a storm — and we're surrounded by enemies. Dr. Dragan is walking on egg shells because of the rapidly changing political climate. He can't avoid getting burned one way or another. During times of war, it seems you have to be someone's lackey just in order to function, otherwise you'll quickly lose your job. I feel that Dr. Dragan's behavior towards me is sincere, decent, and honest. I appreciate that. As a professional, Dr. Dragan stays away from municipal government politics. He's flexible. He certainly understands that life has its ups and downs.

His personal problems are overwhelming. Since I'm a stranger here who's going to leave one day, it's easier for him to confide in me.

Dr. Dragan has four children, one of whom is autistic. He is married to Darija, a Croatian woman, also an anesthesiologist who works with us. They worked in Germany for a long time. They spared no expense in finding a cure for their son. But it was all in vain. Now, the war brought them here, and their fifteen-year-old son is wreaking havoc in their home. He destroys everything that comes into his hands, so he's exhausting the family's emotional and financial resources. Darija is spending her entire pay check on new bedclothes and crockery that the boy keeps destroying. It has been years since they've had a good night's sleep because they never knew when he's going to get up and start throwing all the food out of the fridge or leave the house and start howling.

I suggested that the boy could be accommodated at the Institute for Autistic Children in Serbia. I managed only with difficulty to get in touch with the Director of the newly established Institute for Speech Pathology and Experimental Phonetic Research, who could have found a place for the child. She had never disappointed me, and this time was no exception. She called up two days later to tell me that she found a spot for the boy. It was difficult, but she had managed to pull it off. There are many children with psychological problems now flooding into Serbia, but Serbia could accommodate only some of them. So mentally ill patients are now largely being left to fend for themselves.

When the boy was supposed to leave for Belgrade, Dragan and Darija wept as if he had died. In spite of their personal anguish, and well aware of the conditions that had been imposed on them by the war, they ultimately decided that the child should stay with them. They couldn't bear being separated from him. No one in faraway Belgrade could possibly love him as they did. Besides the problems with their autistic son, their other children suffer frequent asthma attacks. Because of his responsibilities at the hospital, Dr. Dragan can't always be with them. It's also hard to get asthma medication.

I'm going to leave one of these days, just as the other volunteers will. Dr. Dragan and his family, as well as Dr. Savo J., are going to stay right here. Dr. Savo equipped the recovery room with sophisticated equipment that he operates himself. He had obtained his master's degree and then began his doctoral studies in Zagreb just before the war broke out. Now, he doesn't know where he's going to finish his doctorate. It's a normal, logical progression in his profession, and it's an opportunity that he fully deserves. But he's only going to be able to defend his thesis in Belgrade, which will present him with a new dilemma.

As he was confiding these hardships to me, his glasses fogged up. He took them off and wiped them. His eyes were glistening with unshed tears.

"Go to Belgrade," I told him. "You'll be in contact with people who can help you find an advisor for your thesis. Your son can get help there. That'll make things easier until the war ends."

We agreed that I would work every night and that I would only call him when an urgent matter popped up or otherwise in the case of a problem with the equipment. I wanted to give this wonderful doctor, who was bedeviled by more than his fair share of misery, a chance at least to rest.

* * * *

The wounded, the dying, and the dead are arriving from all directions. Bullets have usually ruptured a major artery, so these patients are suffering from severe blood loss. The wounded are pale, and they look as though they no longer have a single drop of blood left in them, but they're still clinging to life. There's no adequate first aid on the battlefield. Or maybe transporting the patients to the hospital takes too long. We anesthesiologists should be on the front line. There we could triage casualties. But the question *Where's the front line?* is ambiguous when people are being killed everywhere. Shells are falling. Mortar attacks wound and maim indiscriminately. And what may sound at first like a distant shell suddenly explodes close by and cuts down everyone in its path. This war, in fact, has no classic "front line" as previous wars have had, where infantry forces engage in hand-to-hand combat. Today, the whole territory is the front line.

We treat many patients with self-inflicted gunshot wounds, which result from fear or inexperience, or which they have deliberately inflicted on themselves in order to avoid having to go into battle again.

One day, they brought in a young man, half of whose head had been blown away: he was dead. Several of his friends, beardless youths between eighteen and twenty years of age who were wearing SMB[9] uniforms, brought him in. They were clutching their caps; they were bespattered with mud; and they were shocked and confused. We started resuscitating the young man according to standard operating procedures. Soon, we were all soaked in blood. When I tried to intubate him, my hand went into his shattered brain. I tried to tell Colonel M. I., the commanding officer, but he paid no attention to me.

"Resuscitate him!" he ordered.

I obeyed his order, so I continued to massage the already lifeless heart. But I asked myself why we were expending resources on what was clearly a lost cause.

Finally, after a full hour of resuscitation, Colonel M. I. said: "That's enough."

Orderlies removed the corpse. The tearful young soldiers accompanied their friend's body in shocked disbelief.

---

9.   SMB refers to the standard olive green-grey uniforms issued by the JNA.

I washed the blood, hair, and brains off my hands and asked the Colonel: "Why did we have to do that? You saw that half his head was gone!"

He was silent for a moment, and then he replied: "Did you see their eyes? They have to know that we're going to fight for each one of them to the bitter end. This is a struggle for their confidence. In this nightmare, they have to trust the medical staff. We must never let them down and we must always give them hope."

Colonel Dr. M. I. surprised me. He was in charge of the medical rescue team that came from the VMA. Something else lies hidden beneath his uniform and his icy, expressionless face. I was too busy to think much either about the depressing incident or the Colonel's wise words. But I know he cares, and I admire and respect his display of constancy and firmness.

4. The Bombardment of Knin

My opinion of Colonel M. I. was confirmed on December 25, 1991, Roman Catholic Christmas, when the first bombardment of Knin suddenly began. Orthodox Christmas is two weeks later, January 7 (according to the Julian calendar), so people were trapped at work instead of family celebrations. It was a cynical choice of timing that was probably made for a propaganda boost.

The likelihood of bombardment had been plaguing us for days beforehand. Knin is situated in a valley. There is no way out except by the main roads. Shellfire and explosions from the surrounding areas reverberate throughout the entire valley. If there are skirmishes around Drniš, then the wounded arrive here in fifteen minutes; it takes about forty minutes to get them here from Zadar. Transportation is well organized for the time being.

At first, the shooting frightened me so much that I wouldn't willingly venture onto the terrace. But as time passed, I got used to the shooting. I became skilled in determining which weapons (judging by their sound) were being used and how far away they were. We're all on edge, so we're hardly able to relax at night or sleep soundly. We're ready to flee at the drop of a hat, but we have no idea of where we can go. We're trapped, doomed from the start. It's slowly grinding us down.

That Christmas Day, we performed two operations with total anesthesia in the Emergency Room on the second floor. We could hear constant cannon fire pounding in the distance. Nightfall was coming and the staff was growing anxious.

In the morning, one of our nurses showed up with her child, who was sick. He had a high fever, and his blood count was very low. He had an enormous number of white blood cells, which indicated anemia. The nurse cried inconsolably. She knew what this could mean.

I tried to calm her down: "There's no absolute evidence that it's leukemia. A series of tests need to be done. There's no certain diagnosis without a biopsy of the bone marrow."

"I know, but I'm still afraid," she replied through her tears.

"Well, even if it is leukemia, it can be cured. He'll get the treatment he needs!" I said, not giving up my optimism.

"How can he be treated, Doctor?" she wept. "There's a war going on! We're cut off from the rest of the world! We don't even have the right medicines. The world's killing us off!" she cried as she became hysterical.

"Go back home," I said. "Stay with your child and try to calm down. We'll manage without you today."

That afternoon I was in the OR with a surgeon. They were bringing in a patient for further observation. The report of small arms fire sounded uncomfortably close.

I was worried. The attending nurses were also upset and they were murmuring among themselves.

"Where's the gunfire coming from?" I asked. "It's been going on all day."

"Don't worry," a colleague replied. "They're fighting around Šibenik...."

He hadn't even completed his sentence when a dreadful whistling sound penetrated the room. A torrent of earth, heaved up by an explosion, surged against the windows of the second floor hallway. A shell had fallen right next to the hospital. Instantly, the lights went out and a siren began blaring from the loudspeaker and echoing through the dark corridors. We were told to stay calm and to remain at our stations. Knin had been bombed. No one was seriously injured. Then we heard the thunderous chords of *March to Drina*.[10] It was surreal.

We ran down the stairs to the tune of *March to Drina*. We had to get to the first floor where the Operating Rooms and Intensive Care Unit were located. Many of us were unaware that we were screaming. Others were hiding their fear behind grim, tightly pursed lips as they hurried along the corridors. We were dazed, colliding, shoving each other out of the way. It was total chaos — every man for himself.

"They bombed the hospital!"

"They're heartless!"

"The Croats are merciless!"

We were whispering among ourselves in disbelief of such deliberate malice. Hospitals and medical centers are supposed to be protected zones. The hospital was clearly marked. It was the only Serbian hospital in this part of Croatia. Before the war, the Cro-

---

10. *March to Drina* (Марш на Дрину), a Serbian patriotic march that was composed by Stanislav Binički and dedicated to a commander of the Serbian Army who had been killed during the Battle of Cer when the Austro-Hungarian Army invaded Serbia at the start of WWI. The victorious Serbian Army meant to liberate the rest of the country from the Austro-Hungarians by marching on to the Drina River, where they intended to confront them. The march remains an anthem of Serbian resistance.

ats were thwarting investment in Serbian regions. So the Serbs took the initiative and built the hospital with the aid of outside donations.

In front of the ICU, we ran into the nurse I had sent home that same morning with her sick child. I was astonished to see her.

"Why did you come back? I asked. "We can make do. Why did you leave your child?!"

"Doctor, I'm a Croat. If I hadn't come today you would have thought that I knew about the bombardment in advance, and that I had deliberately avoided the danger."

She was looking at me with utter candor. She continued: "This way, I'm with my own people. I grew up with them. I love them, so I don't mind if I die with them because they are the best friends I have."

I listened to her with utter astonishment. The dilemmas people face in wartime! Everyone is walking the razor's edge. One decision can potentially be just as dangerous as another because any one of them may end up being a question of life and death.

I ran into the darkened ICU, which was now illuminated solely by the glow of distant fires. The huge windows had no curtains.

The patients were terrified.

"Run! Save your own lives!" they called out. "Give us weapons! You don't know what the Ustaše are capable of doing. They're going to overrun Knin after the bombing raid is over. Get out while you've still got the chance! Don't you get it!?"

"But we have nowhere to go," I answered. "We're here because of you, so we're going to stay here with you."

Nurse Tijana and I start removing the cloth screens from the cubicles in the ICU, and we clambered up to the windows to hang them from the heating pipes. As we were spreading the screens across the windows, we were presenting ourselves as prime targets, but we didn't even think about that at the moment. We simply had to do this. The danger caused our adrenalin to surge. Nurse Tijana, plump yet agile, jumped as nimbly as a doe to the window ledge.

Meanwhile, some nurses were still screaming hysterically. The screaming nurses threatened to transfer their anxiety to everyone around them — we couldn't let that happen. Colonel Dr. M. I. appeared at the door and he ordered them in a strict but calm voice:

"Dress their wounds! Let's go nurse, you … you … and you."

He chose the most hysterical nurses. They looked at him in shock.

"Why now? Why us? Why not get someone else to go!?"

"Do it now!" he continued in a firm but controlled tone. "That's an order! Now!"

The nurses fell silent, and they began pushing patient beds obediently into the corridor in front of the Operating Rooms where the lighting was the best. The work calmed them down and responsibility made them start functioning normally again. That's what I call occupational therapy!

Someone from the crowd shouted: "The multi-national Army — they fucked everything up!"

The Colonel put down the gauze bandage he was holding. His face became stern and he turned to the heckler and said in a loud voice:

"You have to trust the Army!"

I pitied the Colonel because he was defending those who likely didn't deserve to be defended. The Army has begun to disintegrate. It's splintering along the lines of allegiance to the different republics. But the Colonel spoke with the authority of an honest and disciplined soldier. He inspired admiration regardless of whether we believed in what he said or not.

I stick close to people I judged favorably, *i.e.*, in accordance with their deeds. Colonel Dr. M.I. just that kind of person.

5. The Eternal Dilemma

The wounded come in waves. Sometimes ten people — all seriously wounded — are brought to the hospital at once. Grenades and mines are devastating. They sever arms and legs; they maim and cripple young men. Severed limbs or smashed ones that had to be amputated are wrapped in a compress and then thrown in a dumpster. The sound of an electric circular saw buzzing through bones makes my hair stand on end. Medical amputation doesn't pose any serious problems, but tragedy lies in store for the amputee and his family. I'm the child of a war invalid from the Second World War. I'm well acquainted with the problems that arise. Worse, many of these men will never father families.

One young man was cut to pieces by a grenade. He lost both legs up to the knee, his left arm and left eye. When he regained consciousness after having been anesthetized and realized the condition he was in, he spat in my face.

"Why did you wake me up?" he said, lamenting his fate. "My wife died when the war began, my children are alone at home. Who needs me in this condition? Who's going to look after me? Why didn't you just let me die?"

I remained silent. I didn't know what to say. I've never been sadder. His pain was enormous. The walls were crackling with anguish.

I wiped the sputum off my face, but I couldn't wipe away the sorrow.

Later, I learned through friends that my wounded soldier had recovered. It was a real miracle, an act of God. Not only did he survive but he also returned to a relatively normal life. He was also lucky to have a very unusual woman fall in love with him. She was a medical nurse from the VMA. She divorced her first husband and left her children in order to help this poor man. Then in 1995, when I was in Krajina again, I saw him in the village of Ervenik. He was sitting in a wheelchair in front of a local store, talking to friends. Our car slowed down imperceptibly so that I could get a closer look at him, but I didn't want to stop. Why remind him of the past now that he had his life back? That was all I ever could have wished for him. The wheelchair-bound invalid had a bottle of beer at his side. He was throwing his head back as he was laughing with friends. This left me with a misty impression.

But life is never that simple. In 1997, after the first edition of my War Journals was published, he came, prostheses and all, to speak before an audience of 250 people who came to hear his first-hand account of the situation in Krajina, which by then had been lost. This took place at the JNA Cultural Center in Belgrade. My publisher made short introductory remarks. He compared my journals to those of Dr. Pera Stojanović, who was a volunteer during WWI. Then this unfortunate veteran was asked to speak. He took the podium looking as though he had walked out of the pages of our national history. To my utter astonishment, he once again heaped scorn on me for not having let him die. I was utterly nonplussed. The Hippocratic Oath requires us to make every effort to save a life. But what is more important: survival or quality of life? I don't know! It's not for me to judge.

A Wounded Croatian Girl

One night, an ambulance siren roused me from sleep. Sirens are uncommon in wartime. Hearing one means that someone is still fighting for life. The wounded usually don't stand a chance. Death is the norm. As the vehicle approached, the siren grew louder, so it became clear that this was not a typical emergency.

The OR was always ready, so I ran to emergency entrance to await the patient's arrival. The ambulance had already parked. I could see the limp body of a child being carried out. Only when I came closer did I see that it was, in fact, a girl on a blood-soaked sheet. She was pale, almost unconscious. She was immediately taken to the OR. I began inserting a cannula, a thin tube inserted into a vein or body cavity to administer medicine, drain off fluid or insert a surgical instrument.

She did not respond. A bullet had ripped through her left forearm, and another had gone through her left hip. The femoral vein, the largest vein in the pubic symphysis, had been grazed. She was bleeding profusely. She had a vacuous expression on her face and did not respond to questions. When I caressed her head, a spasm of pain and resistance, even anger, contorted the child's face. For a split second, her face expressed terror and profound mistrust. She raised her arm, which just a moment before had been limp, and she slapped my face hard.

The sound of the slap reverberated through the room and it inflicted more pain than seemed possible considering the girl's condition. I was stunned. What had I done?

Soon, a nurse comforted me. She explained the situation: "Doctor, this girl's a Croat from that village where ten people were killed last night. Her mother has been hiding her the whole day. She didn't know who was shooting any more than she knew to whose care her daughter was being entrusted. Everyone's scared. Ordinary Serbs and Croats are scared."

This is what happens when a war starts. Not all Croats support the HDZ, the Croatian nationalist party. Some left their weapons and stood beside their centuries-old Serbian neighbors. That fateful night, a group Serbs and Croats were playing cards — gambling — in the injured girl's home. The mother and her daughter were preparing coffee in the kitchen. Candles cast their warmth on the walls of the room. The cards were flying across the table. The players cried with either delight or disappointment with each new hand.

That was when armed men burst into the room. They raked the players, who didn't even have time to understand what was going on, with machine-gun fire. The innocent card players dropped dead to the dirt floor. Blood, dripping down the walls, made strange, lurid patterns. The mother was in the kitchen, so she escaped the massacre unscathed, but her daughter was wounded by a ricocheting bullet in the corridor. The gunmen were dressed in police uniforms. They came from the night — and melted back into the night without uttering a word.

Soon afterwards, the real Krajina police arrived. They took the dead out to the front yard. Serbs and Croats, neighbors, were now dead! Someone had used the dirtiest trick in the book to provoke a quarrel between Serbs and Croats. Later, the police determined where the perpetrators had stolen the uniforms. Even so, the Serbs at the time neither needed nor were interested in committing such a revolting crime. The perpetrators were never identified, so the toxic atmosphere persists. And it's seething.

The girl and her mother, of course, didn't understand a thing. The mother's instinct was to protect her child, so she didn't want to entrust her to just anyone's care. The girl was bleeding, and by the next day she was almost unconscious. Finally, the mother called the medics from the neighboring Serbian village and they brought the girl to the hospital in the evening. She was pale and exhausted. Her mother trusted no one, so the little girl didn't trust anyone, either — not even the doctors. My mother's heart ached. My older daughter is about the same age as this girl. Who was behind this attack? Her eyes still haunt me.

A doctor from a local hospital, who had honorably remained at his post in Knin, operated on the girl. We already had plenty of experience connecting blood vessels with by-pass procedures. Snipers invariably aim at the major arteries in the neck and groin, so we got to be quite good at mending them. Someone came up with the idea of stopping bleeding from the blood vessels in the neck by compressing them with an ordinary soldier's belt. Many a man's life was saved by this simple technique.

We don't have the necessary instruments for vascular surgery, so our surgeons improvise. Our successes are surprisingly many. We anesthesiologists bear the brunt of post-operative treatment. Maintaining systematic medical care is problematic. Hemorrhagic shock, *i.e.*, a great loss of blood and other bodily fluids, hypoventilation, and the problems associated with them are our greatest concerns. We have problems administering massive transfusions because we lack sufficient reserves of plasma.

After a successful by-pass procedure, the girl was transferred to another department when she was released from Intensive Care. Whenever I had free time, I went to visit my former patients, but I didn't visit this girl. I was afraid of the emptiness in her unfathomable eyes. In moments of solitude, I cried for her in my room, just as I cried for all the children who were victims of this terrible war. Powerless and filled with greater grief than I could bear, I knelt and prayed:

"God, please help all the children ... let them live!"

Our Croatian Colleagues — Prisoners of War

One evening two frostbitten Croatian doctors were brought in from the mountainous Velebit region. They were Serbian prisoners of war. The young doctor who admitted them to the hospital fainted when she saw them. One of the prisoners was a classmate from college. Until quite recently, they had been friends. They went to lectures together, ate lunch and had coffee together, and they went to the same parties. Now, in less than a year's time, they've become enemies.

The young doctor was overcome with emotion. Her friend had specialized in surgery, and now his fingers, on which his career as a surgeon depended, were frostbitten. They called me to resuscitate her, but she didn't need resuscitation. She was completely distraught. She needed consolation.

They found the men tied to a tree high in the mountains. The Croatian doctors wouldn't tell us why their own people had done this to them. We supposed that they had refused to do something that was contrary to medical ethics, so their insane cohorts decided to punish them. They had been cruelly left unprotected in an alpine forest to freeze to death. Weather conditions are harsh on Mt. Velebit during winter, so their hands, feet, ears, and noses ended up getting frostbitten.

One of our patrols found them, then gave them a severe beating after they refused to talk. They were our enemies. Our patrol brought in the bruised and frightened men, who remained silent. They had been beaten by their own soldiers; then they were beaten by ours. Their silence hurt. I could feel it in my eardrums. We didn't speak either. We worked in silence, instead, speechless as we beheld the tragedy of our young prisoners having their fingers amputated. Gone are their dreams of practicing surgery. We quietly lamented their dire fate. After all, they were our medical colleagues. It could just as well have been any one of us. After treating their frostbite, we accommodated them as best as we could.

The next day I entered their room to examine the patients before my regular round of operations. The Croatian doctors looked much better. The older one regarded me with unconcealed hatred, while the younger one slowly got up to drink a cup of water. He tried to grasp the metal cup with the bandaged stumps of his fingers, but it slipped out of his hands and fell to the ground. The jangling metal cup broke the silence and reduced the tension. Reacting reflexively, I looked over the stethoscope I was holding to the chest of another patient I was examining. The young man was staring at me defensively, as if he were expecting to be punished. I was so saddened by his expression that I put my stethoscope down, slowly went to him, and put my hand on his shoulder.

"Calm down. I'll give you water," I said.

I picked up the cup that had rolled under the bed. I washed it with scalding hot water, then waited for it to cool down so that he could drink from it. I gave him warm water to drink. He was still shivering like a frightened animal. My eyes filled with tears again.

"Why are you afraid? You'll be going home soon," I said, trying to calm him down.

His expression changed, and he looked at me kindly as would a child. Tears were running down his cheeks. His colleague, who was watching us, reproached him sternly.

"Why're you bawling in front of her?"

"Let him cry," I protested indignantly. "Leave him alone!"

I left feeling overwhelmed by sadness. I made my regular rounds to see patients in the other rooms, so I finished my daily routine. That evening, I returned to their floor. From the stairs, I heard a racket. It was the clattering of crutches, and it was emanating from a group of wounded Serbian patients who had gathered in front of the Croatian patients' room. They were standing — some on a single leg, others with bandaged heads and hands — and still others whose entire bodies were wrapped in bandages that were bloodstained here and there. They resembled walking mummies. They were grumbling, agitating. I barely managed to plough my way through this pathetic crowd into the room.

One of our doctors who was on duty was standing there with his arms spread wide apart, his face twisted in a grimace of pain, in front of the two terrified Croatian patients, who had been backed up against the wall. Someone had sent a crutch flying in their direction. My colleague, a Serbian doctor, was protecting the Croatian patients from our infuriated wounded soldiers.

It was a ghastly scene. I was choking with rage — so upset that I was unable to speak. The surgeon who was shielding the

Croats suddenly began wheezing. Then collapsed onto the floor. I came to his aid.

I revived him only with difficulty. He had suffered a heart attack, certainly due to stress. He ended up in the coronary unit. He just couldn't endure the insanity of having to defuse an attack by one group of wounded men against another. The absurdity of the situation was representative of life — not only in the hospital, but throughout Krajina, as well.

The next day during our morning staff meeting, it was agreed that the wounded had to be separated. It was difficult to pass judgment on our wounded men, much less lecture them. I sympathize with them. They're barely twenty years old, but they're now without arms, legs, eyes. They had to vent their rage and despair somehow. These young men who have been permanently crippled are the best among us. They can't help but see the Croatian doctors as enemies who are directly responsible for their condition. They attacked them because there wasn't anyone else to attack. How could we have forbidden them to feel anger and indignation? They were maimed in their native land in a civil war, the dirtiest kind of war.

After their convalescence, the Croatian doctors were taken to prison, where they were later exchanged for our soldiers.

Everyday Life

The medical staff takes its meals in the lovely kitchen. Food is often scarce, but when there is food, it's always the same: bread cut into translucently thin slices, sauerkraut, cornmeal porridge, eggs, and broth with a few grains of rice throw in. I was wondering: Where's all that humanitarian aid going? No one has been able to give me a straight answer. For those of us who are healthy, it isn't such a big deal to go half hungry but it's difficult for the wounded, who need to eat well in order to recuperate.

When a young man regains consciousness after having been under anesthesia, and then realizes that he has lost arms, legs, half of his rib cage — he of course gets depressed. As the wounded soldiers calm down, they return to a kind of normalcy. They stop refusing food and they usually start asking for second helpings. As they get stronger, these robust young men want to eat a lot, but we can't provide them with enough food. I steal bread from the kitchen. I save a slice or two of ham or sometimes a fried egg from my plate. I make a sandwich and give half to one for dinner, and then half to another for breakfast.

The medical staff comforts them as well as it can, but we're also depressed. Our daily reality consists of treating once vigorous, handsome young men who have been crippled. Most of them will neither marry nor have children. Their formerly healthy genetic line will end with them. We doctors are tormented as much by this as we are by their wounds. We confront them with the brutal fact that they will simply have to go on living as they are now. We don't hide anything from them. This way, it will be easier for them later. It gives them the strength to show us that, in spite of the difficulties, they will do their best to live up to our expectations. We hope they will bite avidly into the one morsel of life they have left. It's all we can do.

Most of them don't have anyone to bring them food, and it's hard to buy food in Knin. We're cut off from the rest of the country. This region, though, is well known for its production of ham. Somewhere in the hills above Knin, there's a farm that produces smoked ham. The medical staff and war profiteers who were here before us snapped up as much as they could to take back to Serbia. It's shameless that Serbs had carried off the last bit of food from Krajina.

"If ham is the only thing that Krajina can offer, then it might as well disappear," said Dr. Savo J. with a strong note of irony.

I saw it from a completely different angle.

"If I stoop so low as to take from Krajina any material goods under the pretense of helping my own people, then I might as well just disappear."

He shook his head at my stubborn moralizing.

There are no special privileges for working in the OR, either. There is no tea, no milk. People work in silence. All we want is peace and freedom of movement, and a future to go along with it. All this has vanished.

Jelena

We often stay up until dawn. Sometimes we work; other times we listen tensely to the distant sounds of warfare. We count the number of detonations reverberating through the hills. We talk, forgetting about the war for a moment, and we laugh at old jokes and tell new ones. The frontal cortex tries to avoid the madness and horror of war. We also hear terrifying stories.

Jelena lives in the mountains in a solitary house. Her husband and brother-in-law are on the front lines. The unprotected women are alone in their homes with old men and children. Most of the nurses live outside Knin and regularly travel more than fifty kilometers to come to work. Transportation is rarely available since there's a gasoline shortage, so they're forced to find their own way. Those who have to travel only ten to fifteen kilometers in one direction usually walk.

One night, someone knocked on Jelena's door. The unknown visitor didn't respond when asked to identify himself, but instead continued knocking harder. Jelena is robust and audacious, but most of all determined to defend her children. She brought an axe, the only weapon she had, to the door, but even so, she knew she was opening the door at her own risk. She shielded the other members of the household with her body. A man in a uniform stood in the dark outside. Nowadays all uniforms look alike, and everyone is wearing a five-pointed star. There's only one army;

however, the enemy speaks the same language — yet he thinks differently. How are we supposed to distinguish friend from foe? The whites of his eyes were shining in the dark; his teeth gleamed ominously. Jelena was silent; she wasn't sure how many more of them might be in the yard, behind the fence or up in the meadow. She feared the inevitable was about to happen. There was no way out now.

The man didn't speak for a long moment, then in a hardly audible voice he asked:

"What time does the bus leave for Ogulin?"

Jelena was confused, but her answer was cautious:

"It's been a long time since any buses went from here to Ogulin. They rarely go anywhere now. Most often they just go to the cemetery from here."

The visitor was silent for a moment, then turned around and went back into the night without uttering a single word. No one in the house was able to sleep a wink after that. They were all waiting for the other shoe to fall — but nothing happened.

Fog was misting the trees that surrounded Jelena's house when she left for work the next morning. She usually walks to work. There's no other way. As she stepped outside, she took in the bracing air and shuddered as she entered another fog bank — this one of uncertainty. She doesn't look back. That's a bad omen. Now, each time she leaves for the hospital, she fears that it might be her last. On her way — twenty kilometers in each direction — anything can happen. She goes to work in spite of all this. She has to. On the road, she thought about last night's visitor. She wondered who he might have been. The phrase that he used must have been a password. For whom was it? There's no answer. So many different gangs are on the loose. There's no criminal justice system left and none of the laws are being enforced — only madness is left.

The electrical power is more often off than on. Freezers have either been empty for a long time or their contents have spoiled because of the frequent power outages. The night shift doesn't have anything to bring from home for dinner. Most everything in their homes has either already been consumed or been confiscated by roving gangs. Occasionally, a potato turns up or four peppers in a pack. There's no bread. We usually fry what we have. Since there isn't enough to go around, most of us enjoy only the aroma of the food being cooked. Its pervading aroma intensifies our togetherness as well as our desire to survive long enough to see an end to this madness.

We tell stories. From these nocturnal tales, we learn out that most of the hospital staff is in mixed marriages: some Serbian nurses are married to Croatians; other Serbian men are married to Croatian women. Where do the members of mixed marriages belong? Before the dissolution of Yugoslavia, the notion of nationality was considered unimportant when deciding whom to marry. The concepts of *equality* and of *brotherhood and unity* were still current. My husband Miroslav is the issue of just such a marriage. Even so, certain groups, such as Albanians and Bosnian Muslims, in particular, stuck to their own. Their women are forbidden to marry outsiders while the men were allowed to marry women of other nationalities. Their children are, of course, raised as Muslims.

One night, more wounded soldiers were brought in from the battlefield.

"They're bombing us again!" people were shouting.

"Who's bombing whom?"

Everyone fell silent. One nurse leaned against the table and cried.

"Who's bombing us? Is it coming from our side or theirs?" I asked, upset.

At that moment, it wasn't clear who or why anyone would be bombing us.

She remained silent for a long while until she finally lifted her head slowly and spoke:

"What can I tell you, Doctor? I'm a Croat. My parents live in a village where there was an air raid. The Croats were bombing our village! Who's on whose side, Doctor? How do you explain that? We're all heartbroken. We don't know why all this is happening. And what's going to happen to us after the war?"

* * * *

We use telephones only at night. The lines are frequently overloaded during the day, which means it's difficult getting a connection. But at night, when everything calms down, I can call Belgrade first, then Smederevo. Ljuba, my younger daughter, is with my mother in Belgrade, while Marija, her older sister, is attending school in Smederevo. As I had mentioned earlier, I hired Mileva, our maid and nanny, to look after her. This is the kind of help that money just can't buy. I keep their pictures on a small table in my room. Only occasionally do I allow myself to admit how far I really am from my children; how my heart is filled with longing for them; and how dangerous this situation is. I am ashamed of having such fears.

My mother was born in Krajina. My cousins twice-removed live here too. But I've never been to Krajina before. There was no special reason for going, because after WWII my mother's immediate family moved to a village in Slavonia near Podravska Slatina, which is the most beautiful village I've ever seen. All my childhood memories are associated with Slavonia. My grandfather's grave is there. It has vanished now because it was destroyed. After the Croats had systematically forced the Serbs out of Krajina, they destroyed the Serbian and Jewish cemeteries. They wanted to erase every single trace of these people ever having lived in Croatia. Nevertheless, the Slavonian village persists intact in my mind, just as it does in the minds of others who loved it as I did.

It was here in Krajina during WWII that the fascist Ustaše tied my grandmother, who was then seven months pregnant, to a post in the stable by the long black braids of her hair. Then they set fire to the stable. A neighbor, who lived nearby, rescued her from the raging flames. He risked his life going through the rabbit hutches, where he and my grandmother had played as children, to get her out. Then he quickly returned to his company without anyone having noticed his absence.

Later, after WWII, my grandmother testified at his trial that he, a neighbor who was an Ustaša-Blackshirt, had rescued her from certain death. He was then set free and my relatives brought him from Croatia to Serbia and employed him. I remember him. He worked as a security guard in our factory.

My grandmother spent the rest of her life, particularly after my grandfather's death, suffering from post-traumatic stress disorder. My mother also suffered from it. Both of them used to wake up in the middle of the night screaming and sweating feverishly. Inexplicable pains and ailments ravaged their bodies. My grandmother was hospitalized for months at a time. She was subjected to one examination after another, but doctors never succeeded in diagnosing a physical problem. She was constantly reliving the traumatic events she had survived during the war — especially in her dreams — her nightmares. These phantoms left her in peace only after she died.

My mother is also haunted by such memories. As a little girl during the war, she used to take food to her grandfather, who was hiding in a cave. One day as she was going on her way, she came across the bodies of her neighbors, who had been slain. The images of these people — their throats cut, their eyes wide open, their bodies drenched in blood — never left her. I learned how to recognize when she was starting to experience an episode of flashbacks. At such moments, the expression on her face would change and she would withdraw to her room or to the toilet, where she would scream. My mother would become uncommunicative and silent after such unwelcome visitations. Only someone who had experienced similar horrors could understand her.

When I decided to go to Knin, my mother and grandmother were the only ones who did not question my decision. They are the only ones who understand. They were speechless and tearless when they came to see me off. Once, my mother told me that there were people still living in Krajina, ex-Communists, who treated her family, which had been anti-Communist, intolerably. She told me they did not deserve my help since I was the grand-daughter of someone whom they had persecuted. Perhaps she's right, but I can't do anything about it. I did take the Hippocratic Oath, after all.

6. The Republic of Krajina

On December 17, 1991, the Republic of Krajina was pro-claimed. The event took place in a modest assembly hall in the Knin Municipal Building. The chairs in which the audience and participants were seated were as rickety as Krajina's Proclamation of Independence was uncertain.

I didn't realize what creating the Republic of Krajina actually meant. Dr. Savo kept me *au courant*. He explained that independence was a matter of compelling historical significance to the Serbian areas in the newly independent State of Croatia.

An independent State of Croatia? O my God! The last time an independent State of Croatia was formed it was an enthusiastic fascist ally of Hitler during WWII. After having taken Croatia's past into consideration, there is no reason to be optimistic. In recent years, Croatia increased pressure on the Serbs, who were being systematically dismissed from jobs without cause, who were being pressured to convert to Roman Catholicism, and who were then urged to become members of the HDZ, Croatia's nationalist party that was led by Franjo Tuđman. After having declared Croatia's independence, Tuđman outlined a time-tested strategy for ethnic cleansing: one third of the Serbian population would be converted to Roman Catholicism; one third would be expelled; and the remaining third would be executed.

And the Croats started this war! According to Dr. Savo, the Republic of Krajina is simply an attempt to protect Serbs from Croatia's ethnic cleansing policies.

Above Dr. Savo's desk hangs a flag with a double-headed eagle. It's the old Serbian flag which was replaced by the Yugoslav Communist flag (which featured a five-point star) after WWII. What happened to Yugoslavia? My country was Yugoslavia. What would happen to America if some states jeopardized the existence of the entire country by proclaiming independence? An identical scenario is taking place here as both Slovenia and Croatia unilaterally proclaimed independence and seceded from Yugoslavia.

The sounds of the old Serbian anthem *Bože pravde* (*I Impolore You, Divine Justice*) filled the entire assembly hall. Its notes lifted my spirits yet filled my soul with inexplicable anguish.

The President of the Republic of Serbian Krajina, Mile Paspalj, read the Constitution aloud; however, he was unable either to pronounce many of the words or to read the document articulately. It's no wonder because he used to be a chauffeur. I felt sick with shame. The unsuitable choice of a non-university educated person to represent the Republic of Serbian Krajina worried me considerably. The challenges facing this small area, which is already surrounded by enemies and is under attack, are tremendous. I do not know Mile Paspalj personally, but the fact that he did not possess an average level of education speaks for itself. I fear that he's not going to be able to rise to the level of competence the office demands. I'm afraid that he'll end up as someone's puppet.

This situation in Krajina is extremely dangerous for Serbs, who have been forced to seek international support and protection. We need capable leadership, representatives who can communicate effectively with the UN as well as with the rest of the world. Paspalj's substandard reading skills sadly pointed out the obvious: he's not right for the job.

I just want to see Serbs presented in the best possible light in the global political arena. There are educated people in Krajina. Why weren't any of them chosen? Weren't there any other candidates? Under Communist rule, hiring decisions were based on an applicant's political connections instead of his or her education or capabilities. The same principle must be at work here.

I return to the hospital filled with anguish. My knowledge is limited by my prejudices as well as by my desires. All I want is peace!

* * * *

Ten days later. I'm hoping to return to Serbia but the hospital is far from town and I don't even know where the bus station is. I want to work as much as possible, so I didn't go wandering around town to look for it. Besides, no one seems very eager to help me, either. People are tense and preoccupied with their own problems. It's the only way to survive. I finally managed to persuade a junior anesthesiologist, Irina, to drive me to the station so I can buy a one-way ticket out of this physical and psychological hell.

But on the day of my departure, I learn that a group of the wounded is being transported to Belgrade and that they need an escort. The helicopter is flying there one-way. When Colonel M. I. asks me if I can escort the wounded, of course I say yes.

I pack in a hurry while the helicopter makes a rackety landing near the hospital. Medics carry in the wounded on stretchers and place them on the floor of the helicopter, while others, those who are able to do so, sit on the floor. The few civilians who are going to Belgrade take seats on benches near the window.

After boarding, I take a head count and I check everyone's medical documentation. Since I'm leaving, Dr. Savo will never be able to leave the hospital now. It rankles me that Serbia — as well as the rest of the world — is ignoring Krajina's desperate need for adequate and systematic support.

The helicopter rises over the rocky hills. There's snow everywhere. There wasn't any when I first arrived. My doctor's bag is beside me. I begin to feel nauseous as soon as we take off. Exhaustion, disappointment, and melancholy are getting the better of me.

We're flying over Bosnia when I inject Saša, a young man who had been wounded in the leg, with a pain killer. I'm grateful to him because his need for care counteracts my sense of utter uselessness. His face writhes in pain. He grips my hand. He's a Montenegrin from Belgrade. He has three children. This is the second time he has been wounded. A shell fragment lodged itself in his neck the first time. He was lucky because no blood vessels were damaged. Unfortunately, this time a grenade shattered his lower leg.

"Where're they taking us?" whisper the wounded soldiers sitting on the floor.

Their heads must be full of horror stories. After forty minutes of strained silence, someone sitting by the window says, with noticeable relief: "Belgrade! I can see the Obrenovac Power Station."

We land on a helipad near the VMA. Two ambulances are waiting; others are on the way. There are sixteen wounded who have to be taken to different hospitals. I help carry the stretchers together with the pilots, just as any man would. I don't have the faintest idea where my energy is coming from.

We lift a legless woman as the wind blows snow on her. She shivers and draws her arms closer to her body. It's only then that I notice that she's wearing only a polyester blouse and a thin, summer skirt. She doesn't even have a sweater or a coat. I wonder why I didn't notice before.

She looks at me apologetically. "I didn't have enough time to get dressed," she says, her voice trembling.

I suspect she's not telling the truth. She's ashamed to admit she's got nothing to wear. People in Krajina don't wear overcoats because it rarely snows in the coastal areas. I took off my new Canadian coat and draped it over her. I still had a thick sweater on so I wasn't cold. The poor woman's legs had been severed by a grenade. She needed prostheses.

After I send all the patients to their various destinations, I'm completely exhausted. Ready to head home, I reach for the handle of my bag but I can't lift it. I don't have an atom of strength left. Grief is overwhelming me. My colleagues hail a taxi for me. I slump into the seat beside the driver like a sand bag. My disheveled appearance arouses the cab driver. He can tell that I just arrived from a combat zone. He puts his hand on my knee. What an indignity! Enraged, I threaten to slap his face!

* * * *

First, I go to my parents' house in Belgrade, where my Ljuba is staying. She runs into my arms. I kiss her, and I keep kissing and holding her for a long time. My father is wiping away his tears as I greet him. My mother just holds me tightly without saying a word. That same night, I go to my apartment in Smederevo, fifty kilometers away.

Marija, my eldest daughter, is there with Cile. She embraces me but says little. I stroke her soft blonde hair. Her heart beats faster. My two children are very different. Marija is a sensitive girl, always a bit shy. Ljuba is a cheerful, loquacious charmer who attracts everyone's attention.

Cile is tense. He doesn't like the political situation in Serbia, let alone Croatia. As a tax official, he knows well how people are struggling to get by. He doesn't give me many details, but he keeps saying: "It's dangerous… this time it's really dangerous."

* * * *

I put the children to bed. Then I tell Cile about what I saw in Krajina. He caresses me softly. After I fall asleep, I have an odd dream in which I hear grenades exploding in the distance. I also hear the piercing sounds of war planes making bombing runs. I awake. My body is ready to run to the ER and tend to the wounded.

The war has arrived in Serbia with me, and now it's now inhabiting my body.

I return to work at the Clinical Center in Belgrade, where I'm not spared new indignities. My boss asks me in front of everyone to tell him what sex is like on the front lines. I want to slap his face. Instead, I answer angrily: "Next time I go I'll take you with me so you can enjoy sex on the front lines as much as I did!"

But the sarcasm is lost on him. Indifference prevails. There's even a note of mockery directed at the atrocities that are being committed in Krajina. I have to watch myself in order not to lose my self-control — not to mention my sanity.

I jump with terror whenever I hear a streetcar brake and come screeching to a halt. Loud noises remind me of bombs. Belgrade is a big city, so of course there are plenty of loud noises which strain my already overtaxed nerves. Scenes of bloodshed — the eyes of the wounded looking at me — torment my sleep. Then I can't sleep at all. I'm not certain anymore whether everything I see is just in my head or whether I am really seeing it. Krajina haunts my every thought. No one asks me about what is going on over there. No one cares.

I get telephone calls from Knin. My friends need help, which brings me back down to earth. Distant Krajina is suspended in the air, isolated, cut-off from Croatia, and then attacked by it — and abandoned by Serbia. The nurses I used to work with have come to Belgrade with their friends and relatives from Knin to ask me to help them get treatment and therapy at the Medical Center. I take them where they can get help.

I regularly visit the wounded soldiers from Knin we transported to the VMA. Now I take the precaution of dressing smartly to avoid suffering humiliation again at the hands of VMA ambulance drivers. I saw Saša, the Montenegrin soldier, again. A doctor attending him yanked off the gauze clinging to his wound. Saša shrieked in pain. Then the doctor snapped at him: "The tough guy turns yellow when he has to take a little pain!"

I just couldn't let such rudeness pass without comment.

"Shame on you for saying such a thing!" I said. "You're the coward, not him. You've got your ass is parked in a cushy spot but you've got the nerve to lecture a man who left his three children in order to defend people who are under attack? Why don't you go to Knin and brag about your courage to the Ustaše? You disgust me!"

The doctor was staring at me in wide-eyed astonishment. He wasn't expecting a tongue lashing from a lady in a fur coat and a hat.

Meanwhile, the situation in Krajina was growing more complicated and chaotic. I was overwhelmed by fatigue and sadness. Then I came down with a Coxackie virus. I ended up spending March and April 1992 bedridden.

The pay I received while on sick-leave wasn't even enough to cover the fare for a round-trip Belgrade-Smederevo bus ticket. It's a 100 km both ways. Besides being a strain on my budget, the commute is exhausting me. Monetary inflation is getting worse daily. I have to give some serious thought to my future. It's no longer possible for me to continue this way, so I decide to quit my job at the Clinic and go to work at the local hospital in

Smederevo. This way, I can live with my family. Our folklore tradition considers the heart to be the center of the emotions as well as of the life force. I have to follow my heart in order to recover.

Working in the provinces has its shortcomings. I'm barely getting by. As the days pass, I feel as though I'm dying spiritually. One of the few consolations of wartime is that you're better off living in a small town. Everything is close by. You can walk everywhere you have to go. It's even easier to get food. It's a different battlefield, but it's still the same battle.

7. Journey to Kosovo

Hardly a month passed after I began working in Smederevo, when I received orders to go to Kosovo. It was June 1992. Ibrahim Rugova, an Albanian activist in Kosovo, started a rebellion in Priština. He declared Kosovo's independence. This was just one of the countless revolts that Albanians had fomented over the last fifty years. They want an independent Kosovo that will eventually be united with Albania, along with the Albanian areas of Greece and Macedonia in order to create a Greater Albania. Serbs from Kosovo have been subjected to systematic purges over the last one hundred years. Albanians used direct and indirect coercion, including the rape of Serbian women and the burning of Serbian homes. There were even cases where Albanians had rammed bottles into the rectum of male victims. When the Serbs had the temerity to complain, they were further humiliated by the Communist authorities in Serbia. Marshal Tito's Yugoslavia was averse to admitting the existence of any problems which would have destroyed the idyllic image of a multicultural society.

The Albanians have had political autonomy since the early 1970s, and they have the right to use their own language and to organize their own schools.

The Albanian Muslim takeover of Serbian Kosovo — where Priština was Serbia's former capital and where there are about

180 Serbian Orthodox churches dating from the Middle Ages — was, ironically enough, aided and abetted by the Serbs themselves. The purge of Kosovo Serbs has intensified over the past twenty years. More than 50% of the population of Smederevo is composed of Serbs who had been driven out of Kosovo. Everyone in Serbia is taxed the equivalent of one entire day's salary over the course of the year in order to fund Kosovo's development. The Serbs developed businesses, schools, and healthcare facilities. Education spread slowly among the Albanians. Girls are typically married off after their first menstruation. Then they are expected to give birth to all the children they became pregnant with. This results in the Albanians having the highest birthrate in Europe. Families of ten are the norm, and they typically have only one breadwinner. Regardless of the breadwinner's income, there is never enough to provide properly for such a large family.

The differences between Serbs and Albanians are vivid and dramatic: family size, education, women's participation in community activities, and, ultimately, in the economy. The Serbs are having significantly fewer children; women are going to school or working; and Serbian men are better educated than their Albanian counterparts. The education offered in Albania teaches students nothing about the outside world.

A small number of Albanians have been educated outside of Kosovo in Bosnia, Croatia, and Slovenia but they were often able to purchase diplomas through bribery without having acquired the requisite knowledge and skills. Those who studied in Serbia often lacked the necessary Serbian language skills. I personally graduated with Albanian doctors who had received passing grades despite the fact that they were unable to speak any Serbian at all.

Albanian teachers are expected to observe policies strictly so they are quick to accuse Serbs of discrimination. Thus, Kosovo's so-called educated class lacks knowledge as well as skills. So Kosovo remains crippled and, therefore, needs constant assistance from Serbia. We doctors are required to work for a fixed period of time in Kosovo. We have to support the republic's healthcare system.

I worked in Kosovo during my internship. We focused on poor neighborhoods. I made house calls to many Kosovo Serbs. There are huge differences between them and the Serbs from Serbia. One might almost think that these Serbs are actually Albanians, although ethnically they are not. Mixed marriages are rare; most often it was an Albanian man and a Serbian woman. I don't remember a single instance of a Serbian man having married an Albanian woman. Albanian women are permitted to marry only Albanian men. Their social behavior is a result of the two ethnic groups influencing each other. Generally, one may discuss two impoverished ethnic groups with low social status, compared first to the rest of Serbia in particular, and then, more generally, to the rest of Yugoslavia.

We in Serbia hold a somewhat superior attitude toward both Serbs and Albanians from Kosovo. In Serbia, Albanians usually only take the lowest paying jobs because their knowledge of Serbian is so poor. Albanians predominate in crime statistics: theft, murder, rape, and especially drug dealing. They have a well-organized — and dangerous — mafia. Albanians also come from a tribal society where blood vengeance is practiced. Albanians are loyal to each other and they exhibit strong group cohesion because they obey local habits and unwritten laws. But they are strict and can be harsh in dealing with their own people who did not abide by these rules. They don't use the court system to settle disputes. Instead, they take the law into their own hands. Law enforcement is the responsibility of the head of the family.

My father was the head of a large company with 20,000 employees. He was involved in the production of processed meat.

There was plenty of room in the business for unskilled labor. I spent a lot of time with my father at the processing plant, so I became acquainted with several Albanians who worked there. My father was popular with the employees. He was a business leader who invested time in the integration of Albanians into Serbian society. The Albanian men who worked in the plant received assistance. My father was not simply an advisor; he was a man who was willing to help financially when it was necessary. He was chosen as best man for the weddings of several Albanian couples, which our entire family attended. I remember the modest homes these couples had, which consisted of little more than a bed and a table. Later, when these couples had children, they followed my father's advice, so they had no more than three. We participated in the naming ceremonies for the children, who were always given Muslim names.

An old Balkan custom is having the godparents — instead of the parents themselves — choose a name for the newborn child. This is why godparents are respected. My godmother was a German woman who had survived torture and imprisonment in a concentration camp during WWII. Anyone who protested against the Nazi regime risked imprisonment. My father took a managerial position in one such camp that became a displaced person's camp after the war. Many of these women had no place to go, so they decided to stay in Serbia. Gertrauda was a beautiful young woman who stayed and later went on to marry my dad's best friend, who was to became my godfather. There was also a Jewish woman named Martha — Mitzie — who had nowhere to go, so my father decided to help her out and brought her to live with us. She was my nanny, and her influence on my upbringing was crucial to the development of my character.

My father encouraged these people to continue their education as adults. Most of the men advanced rapidly to better paying jobs, such as drivers of garbage trucks, especially on the night shift. My father insisted that women should also continue their education — or learn sewing. I enjoyed these humble families. They were always hospitable when we visited. Some of our Albanian friends bought a bakery and turned it into a profitable business. We liked and respected each other.

So, when asked, I replied that I had no problem traveling to Kosovo. But I did wonder why I was being singled out. There were seven anesthesiologists on the staff. And of all the staff, I had the youngest children, and I had already been to the front. But I got this job because my husband is a respected figure in Serbia as well as in Smederevo. The hospital could have easily refused to hire me. The hospital director did my husband a great favor by giving me a job. Of course, no one else wanted to go to Kosovo.

Cile says that justice doesn't exist, but the battle for justice does. The battle is constant and the only changes that take place result from the efforts of those who take part in the battle.

I left my children again to the care of others. I paid for these services, and then I set out on the journey alone on a bus that departed from the Belgrade terminal.

Priština looks like a provincial Turkish town. The library, which has one thousand minarets, looks like a mosque. The Ramiz Sadiku Sports Arena is also impressive, but these are the only visible signs of culture, be it Asian or European. Everything else — especially the way people behave — is utterly medieval. I'm the only doctor staying in the Grand Park Priština Hotel, so I end up walking to the hospital every day, about four kilometers in each direction. It's a perilous trip because I'm surrounded by Albanians who are not well disposed to Serbs. The political situation is tense. Everyone is anxious and a bit disorganized. I soon understand why my colleagues wouldn't come here.

War is in the air.

I arrive at the hospital and go to the Anesthesiology Clinic. There I see an odd, L-shaped room which consists of two corridors: the shorter one is full of young people who are laughing and sitting in each other's laps, while in the other longer corridor there's a glass cabinet and a couch where three staff members are sitting and speaking Albanian.

One of them approaches me, reaches around me from behind, and easily extends her hand. She doesn't make eye contact with me but curtly says without any preamble: "You're on duty today."

I'm dumbfounded, so I ask a younger doctor: "Who's she, the manager?"

"No, she's his assistant. The manager is on vacation. He's coming back in two weeks. Don't pay any attention to her. She's like that — a little brusque and arrogant — but she's a good anesthesiologist."

I take a second look at her. She's wearing thick chains and multi-colored bangles which are sparkling in the sunlight streaming from the window at the end of the corridor. It's an ostentatious display of wealth in poverty-stricken Kosovo.

I'm confused. It's my first day in the hospital in Priština, and I'm already on duty. I can't even find my way around the hospital yet.

"She doesn't like Serbs. Her husband's one of the leading separatists in Kosovo," a young anesthesiologist says as he looks at me with a sympathetic smile. And, as if he's reading my thoughts, he adds: "We'll show you how to get around, the layout of the Operating Rooms, and the Intensive Care Unit. We'll get you acquainted with regulations and the code of professional conduct. Don't worry! Your colleagues who came here before you weren't any better off."

This introduction neither lessens my annoyance nor diminishes my sense of being unwelcome.

I'm in the Priština Clinical Center. The surgical block appears to be relatively acceptable. At the Center's entrance is the Emergency Room, which is perfectly designed. In addition to essential outpatient departments, there are two Operating Rooms for emergency operations of limited scope. Sometimes we perform as many as twenty surgical procedures there during the night shift. The frequency of patient admissions is much higher at night than during the day. At first I think it's strange, but later I realize that there are many elective surgeries that become urgent at night when management isn't around. The technicians and anesthesiologists are all Albanians and they can be sarcastic and political. They speak Albanian exclusively, and when I politely ask them to please speak Serbo-Croatian, they reply that Priština is Albanian — not Yugoslav — territory.

I'm on duty every other day and I work twenty-eight hour shifts. I get to the hospital in the morning, and then I'm free the next day by 9:00 a.m. Since I don't have enough money for a taxi, I somehow manage to walk — staggering with fatigue — back to my hotel.

About ninety-eight percent of the patients are Albanian. Most of them are either children or old men. Younger people arrive only after fights — which occurred frequently — or traffic accidents. Fights break out when someone draws a knife or a gun in response to a dirty look or an imagined insult. Albanian women rarely come as patients because they are not considered equal to men, so less is invested in women's healthcare. The Albanian women I encounter often beg me not to awaken them from anesthesia because their only purpose in life is giving birth. They're treated like baby-making machines.

The language barrier impedes interaction with all my patients. Either school children or staff members translate for me. The older ones either don't speak Serbo-Croatian or don't want me to help them.

I'm amazed that the majority of patients don't have ID cards, let alone healthcare cards. I also doubt that they're using their real names. They're getting free medical treatment in the Serbian Republic at the Yugoslav government's expense, yet they insist on vilifying the government in word and subverting it in deed.

They frequently bring in patients from private clinics who have a great many complications. They even bring in people who are still wearing their shoes — and completely dressed — straight to the operating table. They roll up the patient's shirt, wash the area to be operated on, and then commence with the operation. I've never seen such things done before! This is a modern OR but the conditions are primitive and unsanitary.

It grieves me the most to see the children. One night they brought in an eighteen-month-old boy. All of his intestines had come out because of an incompetent incision made during an appendicitis operation. They threw a towel over the child, which only partially covered him. The technicians put him on the table even though he was still wearing his baby shirt. I couldn't find a spot to place the stethoscope, nor could I find a free vein to inject him with an anesthetic.

"While I'm treating the patient, the upper parts of his body must be free and reachable for examination and resuscitation," I complained to anyone who would listen.

The Albanian staff reluctantly assented. Afterwards, however, they did not call me for elective surgeries they performed. The technicians worked alone so that I couldn't personally witness their corruption of standard medical procedures. I knew this was taking place. Anyway, I can't change anything in the few weeks I'm going be working here, if anything at all could be changed. The roots of corruption run deep.

The small blond boy who came in with his intestines on a towel was saved because he got the intensive care he needed. I was able to keep him in the recovery room. I took a liking to him immediately. He quickly became my favorite. I drew a smiling clown face with a ballpoint pen on a rubber glove which I inflated. He was charming when he laughed. He had just started to speak, but only in Albanian. A patient in a nearby bed translated for me. I was, in the meantime, also learning Albanian so that I could talk to the boy. We communicated mostly with smiles and grimaces. Whenever I came to the door, he would jump up. I would take him in my arms with all his tubes. I found it surprising that no one came to visit him. For days no one asked about him. One morning, while I was cuddling the boy and speaking tenderly to him, I sensed the presence of the hospital manager looming behind me.

"You like him, Doctor?"

I was startled. The manager, an Albanian, was looking me straight in the eye. I couldn't read his intentions.

"We're playing," I replied. "No one is coming to visit him. He's such a sweet child. I feel sorry for him. He is so tiny and frail. Now we're trying to agree about the language we're going to learn. I only know a smattering of Albanian, and he can't say a word of either Serbian or Albanian."

His answer appalled me: "Why does that surprise you? Families here are large, and they often have more than ten children. One child more or less doesn't much to anyone. You see those two children who arrived brain-dead? They have been here for forty-five days. No one has even asked about them. If a child dies, Allah has taken him. Another child is born. No one mourns the dead, especially not children."

He went on: "You see this child you're holding? He's the seventh in the family. His mother has another baby just a few months old, and she's only twenty. They're in no hurry to come get him. They took him to a private doctor and paid for the operation. Now they can't even think of paying for transportation to Priština. They just can't afford it. If he lives, then it is Allah's will, and they are going to thank him. If he dies, it is again Allah's will, so they're not even going to come back to claim the body. They don't have ID cards — no identity. They fled across the border to escape from Albania and came to Kosovo."

"How is such callousness possible?" I asked.

He shrugged.

"That's the Muslim faith, my dear colleague," he answered softly.

"Tell me one more thing, Doctor. How do you explain the fact that, in terms of percentage, Albanians seek medical treatment more often than Serbs, yet Albanians still complain that they're oppressed by Serbs? Half of the patients here can't even speak Serbo-Croatian, yet they're living in Yugoslavia where they get everything free from the State."

"That's the state policy, Doctor. It's in someone's interest to have such a policy. When there's no more interest, government policy changes," he explained calmly.

"Aren't your Albanian doctors in private practice the worst example of separatism?" I asked. "Because it is directed against your own people. Aren't you aware of the fact that the highest death rate and the highest percentage of complications are found precisely among your patients? You don't even take care of your own people."

As I was speaking, the little boy was touching my face and putting his tiny hand into my mouth. The Hospital Manager was looking gravely out the window. Then he said: "There's nothing that can be done about it. Profiteers always show up during times of crisis. Not even we are spared. But we are both going to be late for our morning meeting."

When I left my little boy, he burst into tears.

The manager said: "Have you thought about taking him with you?"

"I should," I said, half-jokingly. "I have just girls, so a small blond boy would be welcome."

He gave me a scrutinizing look. I don't think he actually thought that I'd adopt a Muslim child. Would they have let me?

"Why are you looking at me like that?" I asked. "Belgrade is a cosmopolitan city. As we speak, Serbia is accepting refugees from all the republics. Everyone is fleeing conflicts between the separatists and the Yugoslav Army. I believe in the spirit and fairness of the Serbian people."

"Do you really believe that?" he asked.

"Not only do I believe it, I know it's true. The Turks were killing us for five hundred years, yet we survived. Then we were being killed off during the First and Second World Wars. Then, inevitably, fifty years later, another war is halving our population again. And yet we're still alive today, and we've been fair to the Albanian people. We Serbs are a head-strong people. Rebelliousness and the will to survive have been woven into our lives. We existed in the past, we exist today, and we are going to be around for a long time to come. History has proven it, my friend."

"In that case, we both have our own misconceptions, my dear colleague," he said, shaking his head sadly. "Let God protect us from each other!"

He probably ascribed my patriotism to naiveté or the influence of propaganda. Maybe he knew something I didn't. I even surprised myself with my sudden tirade. This was new for me. I've been dejected for a long time. I'm disappointed with my own people because personal problems are affecting me. But now, when I encounter obvious injustice towards Serbs, I realize their attitude will prevail unless we stand up for ourselves.

I'm fighting for the truth. Immigrants from Albania never integrated into Yugoslav society, nor did they ever want to. The truth is that Albanians are systematically expelling Serbs from Kosovo.

What Serbs need in order to survive here is faith in themselves. And it is precisely this self-confidence that the world media is bent on destroying. It would be difficult to survive in the turbulent Balkans if I didn't believe my own words. We in the Balkans are all a bit beguiled by our own perceptions of reality.

Staying here with me are nine young men and women from all parts of Yugoslavia who are participating in an open competition for specialization. I doubt that they will stay here any longer than they have to because they haven't been offered any incentives. Evenings, they're not even allowed the freedom of movement to go into town. It's simply so dangerous that they're forbidden to go out. Any possible future career for non-Albanians in Kosovo is completely out of the question.

A new manager, an Albanian as well, arrived on Monday. We both did our medical training in Belgrade at the VMA. He proved to be an outstanding physician and it was a real pleasure to work with him. But it's plain to see that there aren't any anesthesiologists in the whole surgical block besides me who are Serbian.

My Albanian Muslim colleague and I said good-bye at the door of the conference room where the staff meeting is held every morning.

Neither of us are Yugoslavs anymore.

* * * *

When I return to the hotel after I get off duty, I take a shower and then sleep until noon. Then I hurry to the hotel dining room where I have lunch. I generally eat alone because the hotel is empty at the time. My daily allowance is so small that I can't afford to have juice or coffee, so I buy what I need at nearby shops. Sometimes I splurge on a bottle of Coca Cola. The reason for my parsimoniousness is this: My salary was cut after I returned to Smederevo from Belgrade, so I had to watch every penny. My stay in Priština had increased my expenses because I had to pay a woman to cook and clean for the children as well as to take care of them. Cile could not take the responsibility because his job seemed to require his presence twenty-four hours a day.

I went out one evening for a short walk down the middle of the promenade on Priština's main street. There I heard the laughter of men. When I turned around, I saw that a large groups of men in white caps, Albanians — Muslims — had gathered. They were behaving suspiciously — ogling at me, in fact. I was the only woman on the street, so it seemed prudent to turn right around and go back to my hotel room. I thought about how rarely I met any Serbs here. There are fewer and fewer Serbs in Kosovo even though Kosovo had once been the center of the medieval Serbian state. Where do they go for medical treatment? I wonder. I'm not satisfied with the logical answer that suggests itself, so I deny it.

In June, after I had spent an exhausting day on duty, I went to bed in my room at the Grand Park Hotel Priština, as I usually did, at 10:00 a.m. At 1:30 p.m., I was awakened by the familiar sounds of detonations from a battlefield and by the sound of low-flying aircraft sweeping across the rooftops. There was a stampede down the hotel corridors. No one from the hotel staff bother to call me. I was wondering what was going on.

I heard shouting outside.

"The Republic of Kosovo! The Republic of Kosovo!"

I didn't feel like getting dressed. I was just glad that it was taking place while I was asleep instead of while I was awake. Later, the radio announced that Ibrahim Rugova was holding an Assembly to proclaim Kosovo's secession from Serbia, and that violence had erupted. That was the reason for the rioting.

I didn't care anymore. I felt tired and sluggish, so I just went back to sleep.

When I awoke that evening, there was silence — the calm following a storm.

No one mentioned the riots the next day at the hospital. I learned not to ask any questions. The people around me are just as frightened as I am. They don't know the answer any more than I do. The atmosphere was tense because everyone was suspicious of everyone else. The hospital staff is of mixed nationalities (Serbs and Albanians). The family members of many separatists are working here, too. Expressing an opinion in public, no matter which side it may favor, could be dangerous. The dark streets I have to take to walk to and from the hospital are fraught with hazards. Kidnappings are frequent but they're never investigated. Serbs are disappearing.

A shroud of silence envelops the hospital. Mercifully, no one has been injured. The Army and the demonstrators didn't clash this time.

* * * *

Two weeks later, I took a bus straight out of Priština.

Even though I have Albanian friends in Belgrade, I have to admit that what I saw in Kosovo bore no resemblance to civilized European society. Now, the remarks Cile made whenever he returned from business trips to Kosovo come to mind: "The Serbs stopped the Turkish invasion of Europe in 1389 in Kosovo. That battle killed off 70% of the Serbian population of adult men. When the Turks returned seventy years later, they managed to enslave Serbia, and Bosnia-Herzegovina. They stayed for almost five hundred years. They instituted the law of *droit du seigneur*,[11] which intermingled Turkish blood with Serbian."

---

11. *droit du seigneur*, a medieval privilege granted to lords who had to right to sleep with any bride who was being married in their dominions on her wedding night.

The Yugoslav novelist, Ivo Andrić, wrote about relations between Muslims and Serbs in his novel *Bridge on the Drina*, for which he received the Nobel Prize for Literature in 1961. During this period, Serbian janissaries formed the core of today's Muslims in Bosnia-Herzegovina. Serbs organized resistance to the Muslims, and instigated several well-known uprisings in order to reclaim their independence. They drafted their first Constitution in 1835. The Congress of Berlin in 1878 granted Serbia independence, but it did not include Bosnia.

Cile frequently spoke of the great betrayal of Kosovo-Metohija[12] that is seldom mentioned. Metohija means *church-owned lands* in Greek. The Serbian Orthodox Church is the core property owner of Kosovo-Metohija. Cile says that Kosovo-Metohija's records of property ownership are hundreds years old, and that the Serbian Orthodox Church still remains the legitimate owner.

Tito and the Communist Party inflicted a great deal of harm on the Church and its property after World War II. During that war, Albania was annexed by the Italians, then later by the Germans, who killed over 100,000 Serbs in Kosovo-Metohija and expelled over 150,000. When Tito established Communist Yugoslavia at the war's end, he banned Serbian refugees who had fled Albanian terror from returning to Kosovo. Then he allowed 400,000 Albanians to migrate to Kosovo from Albania. And they just kept coming.

The tense work environment and my many responsibilities in Priština had exhausted me, so I fell asleep on the bus. I couldn't sort out all the things I felt. I slept uneasily until I awoke in turmoil when the bus finally arrived in Belgrade. Miroslav was

---

12. *Kosovo-Metohija*, the full name of the Serbian province of Kosovo.

there waiting for me. I couldn't wait to see my children. I threw myself into his arms and cried.

The next day I was back at work in the hospital in Smederevo.

8. The Association of Disabled War Veterans

In October 1992, we established the Association of Disabled War Veterans in Smederevo. I'm on the Executive Committee; however, my interest lies exclusively with permanently disabled veterans. By arrangement with the hospital director, we established a shelter for psychologically traumatized and mentally-handicapped veterans who had returned from the battlefield. Our psychologist took on a huge burden. All of these men remain traumatized. Two tried to kill themselves with explosives; later, six others tried to hang themselves.

The general mobilization found the Serbian population unprepared. Even though separatists in Slovenia, Croatia, and Bosnia-Herzegovina had started the war, no one in Serbia is willing to go fight. We receive little official information about the separatist wars. We learn the most about what is going on from the refugees who are flooding into Serbia.

Those who are mobilized have to leave their jobs and families to don Yugoslav National Army (JNA) uniforms. They are given a rifle and sent to Croatia to defend Yugoslavia from the separatist enemy.

The command structure is neither clear nor coordinated. The Yugoslav Army is internally divided. No one has a clear picture of what Croatian and Muslim officers think about attacks against their own armies. The JNA is itself riven by chaos, so it issues many inscrutable orders. The Yugoslav Army is disintegrating as Serbia is calling for a general mobilization. Officers from Slovenia, Croatia, and Bosnia are deserting the JNA daily. Chaos reigns throughout the chain of command. There were instances where one officer would command the Army to take over a certain territory; then another officer would order the Army to withdraw and surrender it to the separatists. Such contradictory commands formed the environment in which young men were fighting and dying. Militias composed of men who have no military training are being formed by all sides. Innocent people are being killed. Yugoslavia is dying with each and every one of them.

When survivors and refugees arrive in Serbia, they are angry and disappointed with the political leadership. On the one hand, many men who have been mobilized by the JNA suffered physical injuries; on the other hand, they have all been psychologically traumatized. Most Serbs protest. Parents began hiding draft-aged sons. A tidal wave of automobiles filled with young, able-bodied men who are refusing to fight for Yugoslavia is flowing out of the country.

Some politicians organized columns of women to lie on the railroad tracks in front of trains that were packed with young recruits who were being shipped off to fight the separatists. The chaos is indescribable. The media doesn't cover it so it vanishes from everyday conversation. Verbal aggression and protest are everywhere evident.

The people who dodge mobilization don't mince words with those who have decided to fight. Serbia has become internally divided and worst of all no one gives any thought to either the injured or to the families of those who have been killed.

We organized on behalf of the families of those who had been killed. We petitioned the government to compensate these families for their losses; we befriended them and we offered them help. We weren't going to let them be forgotten.

The Smederevo municipal government reacted promptly and correctly. The son of the President of the City Council is serving on the front lines. The President has not used his influence to keep his son out of harm's way, even though he is surely in a position to have done so. He too realized that his son had changed after his return, so he lent us his whole-hearted support.

Companies where the killed and wounded had worked before the war followed the city's example, with SARTID 1913[13] leading the way. The dead could not come back, of course, and no one could give a permanently disabled veteran as much help as was needed. These men are a harrowing rebuke to all wars. All we can really do is help them accept their lives such as they are.

Many men from Smederevo have been mobilized. The dead and the wounded returned home quickly. People are shocked. The municipal authorities, along with my husband Miroslav, spearheaded an effort to mitigate the impression that the government was turning its back on these JNA soldiers. Miroslav traveled with a municipal delegation to Negoslavci in Croatia. There, they were attacked by shellfire. They managed to find refuge in a cellar which soon afterward was filled with earth after another shell exploded nearby. Miroslav was so angry with the authorities after he returned that he immediately bought warm, home-spun sheepskin overcoats for soldiers who were serving on the front. He learned from an inexperienced doctor, a colleague of mine who had been sent to the front lines to do the most difficult of jobs, that the outpatient department was short of medicine and equipment. So I was instructed to procure everything that was needed to fully provision one casualty ward. I also have to find a way to ship these supplies as soon as possible. I went to the hospital dispensary to get medicine and equipment, but I was told that the hospital couldn't contribute any medicine

---

13. SARTID 1913, a steel mill based in Smederevo, which was established in 1913.

at all from its own stores because it was forbidden to send medical aid to Serbs outside of Serbia.

The International Red Cross — together with the United Nations — had forbidden aid to be sent to Serbs outside of Serbia. This is shocking and incredible news, but it isn't an insurmountable barrier. I immediately went to private pharmacies where I purchased medicines and medical equipment as a private individual. I packed everything into the trunk of a car and had it delivered to our young men who had been mobilized in Croatia. The authorities could arrest me now for breaking the rules, but I did swear to uphold the Hippocratic Oath, which means that I have to help those who have been wounded. I don't have time to ponder why the Red Cross isn't honoring the Oath. There's too much to do.

On several occasions, young men on active duty have gathered with their families in front of Smederevo City Hall to protest the war. They want the authorities to answer their numerous questions. The most important is: *Why are we being sent to war when the authorities claim that Serbia isn't at war?* Men were sent to the front where they were either killed or wounded, but these wounded soldiers aren't considered disabled veterans because Serbia is not at war?! Their military ID cards class them all as volunteers, but they were forcibly mobilized. They aren't volunteers in any sense of the word. We all know that. Many, who were about to be mobilized, just got into their cars or took planes or trains to flee the country. Families that had money to hide their sons from the mobilization did so. The poor, who have nowhere to hide, go to war just as the poor have gone to fight many a war since the beginning of time.

The other problem is that all the soldiers who did see combat have first-hand knowledge of the reigning state of anarchy. To put it simply, they encountered complete chaos. No one knows what the JNA is going to do and no one knows who's in charge because the chain of command is breaking down. This has resulted in JNA soldiers suffering casualties from friendly fire, as was the case when these soldiers were bombed by their own Air Force. There are no clear battle plans and there is no clear military objective. The government says the objective is to protect Serbs in areas where they've come under attack, but no one knows what the final strategy is. This state of affairs only serves to encourage the formation of paramilitary groups. Discipline among JNA troops is poor, and many mistakes were made that have later proved to be costly. The crumbling national establishment is unable to answer these crucial questions and local governments remain silent — but the JNA soldiers still want answers.

Miroslav is in the vanguard of those who demand that the highest authorities articulate their policy, goals, and strategy. I'm afraid for his life because of his outspokenness. I begged him to calm down and not to compromise himself by speaking out against Slobodan Milošević. I begged him not to call Milošević a traitor, but Miroslav isn't a man who can be easily influenced. He has his own opinions, and he always stands behind them.

I often receive telephone death threats against his life. Unfamiliar voices tell me to buy a coffin and wait for his dead body to arrive. At first, these threats were ominous. I didn't dare mention them to Miroslav because he already knew he was in danger. Then one morning, I heard someone breaking into our apartment. When I ran into the corridor, I found a man wearing a mask who was holding a weapon in his hand. Without thinking, I jumped on him because he was right in front of the children's bedroom, where they were asleep. Miroslav heard the commotion and came running out of the bedroom in his underwear. Meanwhile, the children were awakened and they started crying. The masked man fled through the broken door. After this episode, we installed a metal security gate on the inner part of the door so that it wouldn't be so easy to break in.

I wanted to file a police report but Miroslav advised me not to do so because he suspected that it was the police in fact who were threatening his life. He had once quarreled with the chief of police. The dispute stemmed from long-standing disagreements that began years ago when Miroslav was a public defender and the current chief of police was a judge. Miroslav was not involved in politics but the chief of police was. Cliques can be found everywhere but Miroslav doesn't belong to any of them. I myself can't believe that the police, who are supposed to protect us, are actually organizing a campaign of death threats and break-ins. As a doctor, I've often worked closely with the police. We would meet during investigations and we would also coordinate the transport of patients. I also taught them first aid in official training classes. Why would they terrorize my children? Miroslav is their stepfather; he's the breadwinner. I have to do something. I think of finding people whom I trust in the police force. I'm willing to do anything to protect my family.

One night, I was standing by the window when I saw a man get into our car and drive it away. He just up and stole it right before my eyes! I quickly awoke Miroslav, who had just fallen asleep. I was upset. I riled him from sleep and told him what had happened. He reluctantly got up, walked over to the window, took a look at the empty space in the parking lot where our car had been parked, and then came back to bed. He said: "My dear, it's 3:00 a.m. The guy who stole our car is already gone and on his way to wherever he's going. The police can't do anything about it now, and they can't do anything about it in the morning. I have a difficult day ahead of me tomorrow. If I were to go to the police now, then I'd be dead on my feet tomorrow. Maybe that's why that guy stole our car. If I suppose correctly, the car will be parked in the same spot tomorrow, and it won't have a scratch on it."

Miroslav went back to sleep but I couldn't. I was too frightened.

"We're at war," he used to say. "It doesn't matter what official designation this idiot gives it — we're at war. And things are going to get worse before they get better. Yugoslavia is breaking up and we're going to be confined to one republic. Serbia is going to be divided up into cantons. You'll see Smederevo become a separate canton. It'll start on Serbia's border with the Drina. Later, things will take their own course.

"During this initial phase, chaos is concealing the privatization of Yugoslavia and Serbia. This idiot, Milošević, is passing himself off as a Communist but he's the one who's privatizing Yugoslavia and Serbia at the behest of the United States.

"All public property, as well as anything that was once state property, is going to lose its value overnight. Then a public auction is going be held to sell off the assets. That's when Milošević's relatives and cronies are going to buy it all up for pennies on the dollar. You and I haven't got the money to buy a one-family apartment, even though we spent years getting an education and working like draft horses. They're going to buy up our factories with our own money, cut us out of the picture, and then they're going to make huge profits.

"But this won't last long," he added. "People like them only know how to lose money and property. They're incapable of managing financial matters, so foreigners will come to the rescue. Then they're going to buy up those factories at bargain prices and take over. Before that happens, though, the country will be reduced to ruins so that people will be forced to work for free.

"Ah, my blood pressure jumps whenever I talk about this stuff. I'm overwhelmed. Sarah, I'm certain that they're going to kill me. I assess all the property that's sold, and every day I have to prepare two sets of documentation: one for the buyer and the seller; the other for myself. They want me to assess these properties at a very low valuation — even if I disagree. If I'm being forced to accept their conditions, then I want the truth to be known. It's fraud."

He looked at me tenderly and said: "You have children, so I don't want to get you involved. I don't want to put you through even more pain than you've already experienced. We should get a divorce. You have to get away from me. You and your children don't have to either bear my cross or pay the price."

* * * *

Seven hundred people came to the Cultural Center in Smederevo for the inaugural meeting of the Association of Disabled Veterans. The hall was packed, and people were standing in the lobby because others were already sitting on the steps between the rows of seats.

The soldiers want answers. They demand that their service be recognized as well as compensation be paid for their disabilities. They want acknowledgement of the sacrifices they've made. A murmur of protest arises from the crowded hall. There's palpable tension in the air. It feels as though a screaming match might erupt at any moment.

Disagreements and divisions have unfortunately plagued the Serbs throughout history. This evening was no different. There was no chance of these disabled veterans receiving any aid. One after another, official speakers came to the platform and spoke of the dangers of the front. They spoke of the need to acknowledge the volunteers' efforts, achievements, and sacrifices. I felt sick at heart. What had they really done? They fought a battle which we lost! I don't know how we lost, whether it was their fault or their commander's, but we had nevertheless lost. There's a huge difference between those who went to the front and those who fled the country to avoid conscription. It's indisputable, but it's also true that no matter how significant their efforts and sacrifices had been, and no matter how much time and effort I had exerted in

Krajina, we didn't contribute much to the substantial improvement of living conditions for the people we were supposed to defend. We hadn't even lived up to our own expectations.

That was the reason I took the floor. I said: "I would like to welcome all the soldiers who took part in this miserable war. It seems to me that you have misunderstood the purpose of this gathering. We did not gather here to hand out medals for bravery or to choose the best among us. Yugoslavia is losing this war and no one gives medals for lost wars. We have gathered here to help the disabled veterans and to help the families of those who came back in coffins. We didn't gather here to be divided against one another or to struggle with the authorities in order to obtain political power. We have gathered here to find the best way to help the weakest among us. The government may forget, but we must never forget either the disabled veterans or the dead. Long live humanity, ladies and gentlemen. Let's establish an Association that is going to help the weakest among us. Then, after that, we can deal with the authorities."

Ominous silence reigned. I felt the walls closing in on me. My footsteps echoed in deadly silence as I left the stage and returned to my seat in the first row. The President of the Executive Committee of the municipality, his face reddening with repressed fury, his eyes wide open, was whispering something to my husband. He was saying that I had been undiplomatic to mention such things.

Silence oppressed us for a moment. No one dared make the slightest move. Then one veteran pounced onto the stage, grabbed the microphone, and pointed at me and started roaring:

"Listen, Doctor, if you weren't a woman, I would beat the living daylights out of you. That's how desperate, disappointed, and furious I am. I can see that you too are desperate because of all of our casualties. Comrades, fighters! The Doctor's damn right! We have to help each other and establish this Association to help the disabled vets and the families of those who really need help while their boys are on the front line.

"The government isn't giving us enough support, so we have to take charge. We can settle accounts with the government later. Thank you, Doctor, for the shock therapy."

The meeting room resounded with thunderous applause. I had to stand but I couldn't see anything through my tears.

The next morning, the newspaper appeared with the headline: *How Quickly the Government Forgets*. And the article featured a photograph of me. The struggle has begun. The media is paying attention to us.

Radio stations start interviewing us, and frequently at that.

The White Eagles

They would bring us wounded soldiers from the front whose uniforms bore different insignias. They ranged from the five-pointed star of the Yugoslav flag to the double-headed eagle of the Serbian flag. But once their bloody uniforms were torn off, these soldiers were all the same. The same motives, the same youth, and the same goal: they came to help their people who were being killed on their own centuries-old territories. We doctors had to concentrate on their injuries. Our patients were members of all the different parties to this war.

An apolitical attitude characterized the Association of Disabled Veterans. Consequently, my patients included members of Vojislav Šešelj's *White Eagles*. One of them came to me after having spent a year in Bosnia. His physique was youthful, but his face resembled that of a much older man. Unpleasant spasms of pain had distorted and wrinkled his face. His eyes were sunken. His abundant hair had grown prematurely grey. Scars furrowed his hands, which he pressed together to prevent them from trembling uncontrollably.

"Doctor, I heard you speak on the radio, so I had to come to see you," he said. "I hope you don't mind. I had to talk to someone who can understand what's tormenting me. Now please listen to me...."

He stood up abruptly, then started walking in circles around the living room.

"Excuse me, please! I can't sit down," he muttered. "It's easier when I pace. Then it feels like I'm getting rid of these damn memories."

"Let's take a walk along the quay," I said. "No one's there at this time of night, so you can even scream if you feel like it."

"Let's go!" he said, agreeing immediately.

The streets were almost deserted. It was a late December night and it was cold enough to make our teeth chatter. The two of us walked through the park along the Danube. Lights cast the shadows of anchored vessels onto the promenade.

He told me his story as we walked.

"We went on a reconnaissance mission through Serbian villages. Our job was to eliminate any remaining enemy soldiers and to deactivate booby traps and mines. We were always cautious. You have to be systematic. We're experts. We've seen everything — dead old men and children. In the forest, we sometimes came across the beheaded bodies of our soldiers. Mujahedin — Muslim holy warriors — decapitated them to frighten people. Their treachery only enraged us.

"One day, we cautiously approached a small group of isolated houses. There was smoke rising from one of them. The enemy was either still there or had just recently left. We reloaded our weapons and entered the house. I was petrified when I saw the terrible sight that was awaiting us. We've seen plenty of horrible scenes since the war began, but we hadn't seen anything quite like this. I have no words to describe it. There was a spit over a dying fire. The smoke from this evil fire was rising into the sky.

There was a man impaled on the spit. His abdomen had been ripped open. It was *Murad's incision*[14] and all his entrails were hanging out, and some had fallen into the ashes. Blood was still oozing, and the poor man was still alive. His eyes were swollen and his skin, a red-black color, was cracked all over.

He whispered: "If you're Serbs... if you've got a heart ... kill me!"

"Who did this to you!?" we asked.

"Mujahedin," he barely managed to whisper. "We had to read his lips. Then I fired a whole magazine of bullets into him because I was afraid that one bullet wasn't going to kill him. I wanted to be sure that he was dead so that he wouldn't suffer any more."

"Aaaaaaaaaaaaaaaaaaaaaaaa!!!" The young man roared. "I'll spend the rest of my life hunting you green[15] bastards down! I remember the sun was setting behind a mountain, and orange gleams of light were mingling with the falling night. I was roaring and shooting into the sky: *God, are you there?!*"

His roar echoed eerily among the dark, empty houses. He knelt down and began scraping the frozen ground with his bare hands. Then in sorrow and in anger, he threw dirt on his head. After a few minutes, he sighed heavily, and continued his story.

"We dug a grave and buried him. We made a cross from the stakes of a picket fence. We used charcoal from a piece of burnt wood to write on a board in capital letters: A SERB. We said a prayer at his grave, and we made a vow: *We're going to avenge*

---

14. *Murad's incision* is an incision made from the navel to the throat in order to disembowel a human being. The name arises from the Ottoman practice. The eponymous Murad was the leader of Ottoman forces during the Battle of Kosovo in 1389.

15. *green* is the color favored by mujahedin.

your death if it takes us as long as we live. We are going to send all those mujahedeen to Allah!

"Doctor, I dream about his swollen eyes, and I always hear his words: *If you're Serbs, if you've got a heart.... kill me....* Can you believe that a Serb asked me to put him out of his misery?"

His anguish was physically painful to me, as well.

He wiped his hands on his knees and whispered: "It's like drug addiction. You know that it's not good for you, but you can't do without it any more. I can't pull myself together. I'm haunted. I feel sorry for those people. We know how much they need our help no matter how insignificant our help is. Animals that kill with such diabolical pleasure should be wiped off the face of the earth. We have to exact revenge, otherwise they're just going to keep on killing."

He sat down on the banks of the Danube. He covered his face with his hands. I sat down as well. We were silent. Only our sniffling could be heard. We were carried away by a kind of tranquility. The woods cast their dark shadows on the far side of the Danube. The bridge leading to Kovin was shimmering in the distance. We rose like a pair of shadows. I slapped him on the back. I couldn't see his eyes, but tears were trickling down his nose. Arm in arm as elderly couples do, we made our way quietly back to town. Our footfalls were echoing as we walked along the promenade next to the river. The pain had erupted and escaped from our bodies just as lava that shoots forth from a volcano. We were empty.

We reached my apartment building.

"I'm sorry, Doctor..." he said, turning around and receding into the darkness.

Then he stopped and added: "If you were to ask me whether I had also killed an innocent person or had robbed his house, rest assured that the only person I ever killed was that Serb. I once took a pair of gold earrings from an abandoned house. They probably fell out of a plastic bag that the owners or robbers had taken with them. I gave them to my wife. They weren't blood-stained. There, I got it off my chest. Maybe I'll just throw those earrings in the street for someone to find. I don't want anything from there. I didn't want these memories either. But they aren't so easy to get rid of."

"Good-bye!" I called to the shadows as he vanished.

I never saw him again.

9. Back to the Front in Krajina

The Association of Disabled Veterans organized a humanitarian concert. All of the income has been earmarked to support the wounded veterans. Olja Spasojević and her girl band sang to the accompaniment of the JNA Orchestra. After the concert, a new notice arrived from the Ministry of Health stating that I was being sent back to the front lines. It was Thursday. On Saturday morning one group was scheduled to leave for Krajina. Where are they going? Glina? Knin? Knin seems to have its quota. No one really knows.

Not one person from the hospital in Smederevo responded to the appeal. The chief surgeon, who was supposed to set an example and organize the departure of volunteers, promised publicly that he would be the first to go to Krajina. He later retracted his offer. The hospital director made a conspicuous show of coming directly to me with the notice. The pressure was on. There were eight anesthesiologists in our department but the Director spoke directly to me instead of addressing the others.

Miroslav was agitated and distracted. The political pressure on him was growing. He complained continually that the police were following him and that he was in real danger, so I tried to find people I could trust to help him. There are always good and bad people. The trouble is that we're at war and there's constant pressure to take care of yourself and your family first. There's no energy left for the welfare of others. In fact, no one knows any longer what goodness is. The word *justice* has come to mean the ability to survive under constantly changing conditions. For that reason, I can't be sure that my connections in the police department are actually working on Miroslav and my behalf. Nevertheless, I have to trust someone. My dilemma about returning to Krajina was resolved with the help of my contacts in the police department, as well as after discussions with Miroslav. The fact that I'm going to Krajina again will strengthen my husband's position. It may even save his life, which seems to be dangling by a thread. He knows that my departure can help him, but he doesn't like the idea of my being separated from my daughters and of my being exposed once again to danger. I'm afraid for Miroslav just as I'm afraid for myself. Miroslav wants to bear his fate alone. He doesn't want to involve me or my children. The price has become too high. He wants to get divorced as soon as I return. I refused to discuss it at that particular moment, but I know the situation is grave. We did, however, arrange some of the details in advance.

Whatever excitement I may have felt before leaving quickly vanished. The pain and gravity of the situation puts me into a trance, so I'm unable to respond to people who are speculating about my motives. If only they knew how high the stakes are, they never would have opened their mouths in the first place. I feel as though I've grown old in a matter of days. I leave the children with their nanny Mileva, who used to look after them while I was at work. And I give her money for food. I leave my life savings with my neighbor Nada to hold for my children just in case something should happen to me.

The second parting is far more painful than the first. Marija, my older daughter looks at me, and says: "Mom, don't worry. Everything is going to be all right. You'll come back. If I was bigger, I'd go with you. They need you more there than here."

Ljuba, who is four, embraces me.

"Heaven help you!" she said. "Save some child like me and bring her here so that we can protect her from the war."

I embrace them but say nothing. My children are better than I am! There is no book in the world from which they could have learned more. We had a lesson in honesty and self-sacrifice. They will learn the hard way what life is like in my absence. Let them learn. I want them to be human beings.

Miroslav helped me with my preparations. He tried to comfort me, but I saw tears in his eyes more and more often. He was hiding something from me.

I decide not to call my mother this time. I know she's going to burst into tears. She's been pushed past the breaking point. Only a few days ago, the Croatian Ustaše killed twenty-three young men in Gračac, her native village. French UNPROFOR soldiers allowed them pass through to the Serbian side during the night, where they launched a surprise attack and slaughtered the young men while they were still asleep. They had even cut off their ears and genitals. I thought the French were our friends, but I was wrong. We don't have friends anymore. My mother weeps inconsolably. Four of her nephews were among those who had been slaughtered. All of them were members of the Special Forces. Such villainy is intolerable. I felt a dull but persistent pain in my stomach, and it didn't go away until I finally committed myself to returning to Krajina. Only then did I calm down.

Miroslav and the children took me out for a farewell lunch. I never imagined that it would be our last. That evening, young men from the Association and my journalist friends took me out for a drink. They gave me pencils and reams of writing paper.

"Now you can write to us," they joked.

"Do you intend to go wearing all that gold?" they asked, teasing me deliberately because a few days earlier Miroslav had given me a golden wedding band.

"Thanks for calling it to my attention," I said, smiling. "I'll take the ring off. The Ustaše just might cut off my finger to get it."

Glina

We traveled down an empty road for forty minutes in dense fog before we finally arrived in Belgrade. A black Citroën minibus bearing Glina license plates was already parked in front of the Ministry of Health. It looked like a black panther, ominous and ready to bolt. It seemed as though it could either launch a defense or a deadly attack. The driver, dressed in camouflage, revved the engine, which confirmed my impression of the vehicle's pent up power. He had a grin on his face and his eyes sparkled. I've seen many people like him in this war. They're always on the go and they never stop unless they either lose their last ounce of strength or someone kills them. Stress keeps them highstrung and alert. They're ticking time bombs ready to explode.

Our luggage was already stowed on the minibus, but there were still five empty seats. One of them was mine. Who was going to be sitting in the others? People were scurrying around us. The shops were full. Buses were passing by. The guards from the Ministry checked our ID cards. Dr. Rakić, our Coordinator, came down to the Main Hall. The first news we got wasn't very promising: there was no hospital in Glina. It was a health center built fifty or sixty years ago that has since been converted into a hospital. The Yugoslav government, relying on its fiscal policy, decided to close the health center because it was on Serbian territory. Yugoslavia was not a country beloved by all of its citizens.

Now it's clear that some people regard Yugoslavia as "a prison of nations."[16]

Before the war, about 120 people worked in the Glina Health Center, but now there are about 200 employed there to meet the needs of the entire Banija and Kordun regions. The improvised hospital has no anesthesiologists, so I'm going to be the only one in an area that serves 250,000 people. I'm uneasy about the assignment. Then a surgeon appears who's wearing a pair of black Ray Ban sunglasses and cleated boots. He has, evidently, prepared himself for the rugged mountain terrain. Next comes a general practitioner, a tall, dark, bearded man who had the graceful manners of a writer. There's also a tall, thin ophthalmologist from Niš named Jovan who has already been to Glina. Since he's returning, I reason that can't be as bad as the stories I've heard about it.

We exchange noncommittal smiles while we cautiously size one another up. I can tell they are taken aback because I'm a woman. They don't say a thing, but I can sense their disapproval. It can't be helped. Krajina needs well-trained medical personnel. We all take what we can get. Krajina is in a humiliating situation, trapped as it is between malevolent forces that are tearing it apart. Krajina is the location of a hole in the hull of the sinking ship of state.

The black Citroën takes to the road noiselessly. The road is clear as far as the Bosnian city of Brčko, so there's no indication of a war going on. But as we enter Brčko, we see the flame-blackened walls of one house after another — their windows and rooves blasted out — all reduced to ruins. We look for the hospi-

---

16. *prison of nations*, this was a phrase popularized by the German press in the 1990s to describe Yugoslavia.

tal. I want to see the Director, Dr. Moma Crnić, an amiable doctor whom I met a few months earlier at an anesthesiology seminar at the VMA. We attended the same training sessions there.

The Brčko Hospital is partially damaged. Bullet holes peppered the walls and mortar shells had cratered the court yard. The hospital has been in a state of chronic disrepair for so long that it's now crumbling. Dr. Moma has a shell on display in a glass cabinet. It looks like a grotesque piece of contemporary sculpture. There's an oak branch above an icon of St. Sava that's slanting toward one of the many cracks in the walls of his office. He's no longer the cheerful, carefree charmer I met just a couple of months ago. His attitude now is one of resignation. I can't tell him that most people in Serbia share his sense of resignation, which amounts to a withering view of reality devoid of optimism. He says something typically Serbian, which makes me feel ashamed of these thoughts:

"You know, I feel more at ease now that you are here. At least we're not alone!"

We're certainly not alone. I feel my morale and self-confidence rising, which would be enough for two people. I'm ashamed of those who declined to volunteer to come here, as well as of those who made the cowardly choice to flee the country. There are only a few of us on Krajina's side. Are we enough to ensure victory? Perhaps. The people of Krajina have enough strength and wisdom; what they need now is support. We have to keep our spirits up. I know that we're on the side of right because we're volunteering to help save lives. The staff isn't going to let us leave hungry, so we joined them for a meat and potatoes lunch in the kitchen. They usually prepare food in a soldiers' kettle, so this meal is a special occasion.

"Stop by on your way back so we can eat well again," they joke.

If we're still alive, each one of us privately thought — but no one is going to say anything that might jinx our luck. Judging from the devastation surrounding us and from the explosions that we hear in the distance, this is no joke. It's a war.

Our driver, Pierre (who, true to his commando appearance, is an experienced front line driver), accelerates as soon as we closed the doors. He takes curves at hair-raising speeds. We're dodging sniper fire, he says, and he tells us that hitting a moving target is far more difficult, so we slink as low as we can in our seats and keep quiet.

There's a skinny boy wearing fatigues who is standing on the roadside on the outskirts of Brčko. He's about ten or eleven years old. His alert, vulnerable eyes glimmer under the oversized cap on his head.

"He stops passing trucks," Pierre tells us. "His father was killed about six months ago. A grenade blew him up somewhere in the mountains. They couldn't find enough of him left to put in a coffin. Ever since, the boy's been waiting for his dad to come home. He stops the trucks and looks at each and every driver. He's still looking for his dad."

The boy is unaware of the waking nightmare in which he's living in. He's in denial because he's certain that his father has to come back home. He knows that his father would have never left him. That's why he's been waiting and searching for him for day after day, week after week — for months — because the reality is intolerable. He can stand on the roadside from dawn to dusk. He's not afraid of snipers. Mother Nature is protecting him. Adrenalin and tension armor and shield him.

Tension and fatigue finally exhaust me, so I drift into an uneasy sleep.

We remain silent as our transport vehicle glides down the road. Each one of us is sorting out private thoughts. Behind us, the blazing orb of hot orange sun is setting; ahead of us, the pale moon is rising in the dusky sky. It's peeping timidly above the treetops of a darkening forest, which blends into the curtains of nightfall. Then only the road is visible. We pass shadowy houses where salamanders are burning and around which uniformed men are huddling to keep warm. Armed civilians frequently stop us and ask to see our documents.

"Volunteers! Doctors from Belgrade. Go head!" they say, saluting and waving us through a check point. Much later I came to understand what Belgrade means to them. It's a sanctuary that represents hope and salvation. We represent a bond of goodwill. We're heralds of loyalty and purveyors of aid crucial for their survival. If my colleagues in Serbia could only know how badly these people need us. Simply being here means so much to them.

We finally arrive at the hospital in Glina, where they check our documents again at the reception desk. It's already late at night. The dim hospital lights barely illuminate the hallway. On our way here, we were advised that Glina had neither water nor electricity. The hospital relies on its own generator. There's no welcoming committee. No one knew when we were arriving or whether we would arrive at all. We carry our luggage into a barely functioning elevator and go up to the surgical ward. Nurses emerge from the semi-obscurity to meet and escort us to the empty patients' rooms where we're going to be staying. The men return to the ground floor together, while I stay alone in Room No. 3 next to the OR. A kerosene lamp emits a feeble light. Nurse Radica brings me a wash-basin, so I wash up with water I brought from Smederevo. I change into my nightgown and lie down in the bed, whose little wheels rock back and forth as a boat does. The mattress is coming apart in the middle. I'm exhausted. I try to find a comfortable spot. Then I finally fall into a deep sleep — but not for long.

I'm awakened by howling dogs. Their baying vacillates, at one moment near, at another far. I think about my children. This damned war, I think. I simply had to come. It's my duty as a physician, but I'm still upset about having left my children. I try to bring my mind back to my reality, where my struggle for peace must begin.

Suddenly, I hear a commotion in the corridor. Someone is calling my name. I get up and dress. I have to work right away. A woman has to have a caesarean section. It's a *placenta previa*, a condition in which the placenta partially or wholly blocks the opening to the cervix, and thus interferes with the normal delivery of the baby. This woman is bleeding heavily. The baby is asphyctic and its heartbeat can barely be heard. I put an oxygen mask on its tiny face. I aspirate and then ventilate, and repeat this for five to six minutes. A flush finally returns to its face, and the baby starts crying.

"One more life's been saved," says a surgeon with a charming smile.

Once again I lie sleepless in bed. The darkness and the distant baying of dogs envelopes me. Somewhere far away, I can hear the Serbs changing guard.

* * * *

Morning bursts into the room with the cleaning lady and her broom. The nurses give me slippers to wear outside the OR. I wearily put on my uniform. The nurses show me the ICU, which consists of two rooms with three beds each. These must be rooms for less critical intensive-care patients because none of them have an oxygen supply. The ICU is virtually unequipped.

My work has begun. I'm not intimidated by it. Two of the improvised operating rooms have military anesthetic machines, the kind used in field hospitals. As luck would have it, I'm already familiar with them. They're easy to operate. The oxygen is supplied by canisters because there's no central gas supply, storage or distribution system. I have three anesthetists. Slavica, the forty-seven-year-old ex-wife of the former Minister of Health, is an excellent anesthetist. She's meticulous, hardworking, and knowledgeable. I find her very helpful because she spends all her time at the hospital. Vladimir is also there. He's a Croat from Karlovac whose wife is a Serb from Glina. She's a nurse in our Surgical Ward. They have two small children: the girl suffers from celiac disease; the boy is epileptic. Finding medications and gluten-free food is an on-going difficulty. Their lives are anxiety-ridden because either one or the other child is likely to be sick. From my experience, Vladimir has psychological issues common to mixed marriages. He had to control everything. He came as a freelancer when there were no anesthesiologists in the hospital. He believes he knows a lot, so we often end up arguing over procedures. Since he's been working alone for a year, he has been appointed lead anesthetist, although Slavica is much more competent and hardworking. Then there's the beautiful Lana, the junior anesthetist. She's enthusiastic but still unsure in emergency situations, so she has to be carefully supervised.

Following my resuscitation of the baby last the night, I learn that there aren't any resuscitation kits, so I immediately start gathering the necessary instruments with Slavica, and we assemble two kits: one for children; the other for adults. We don't have adequate boxes, so we put the kits into two separate, large plastic bags. There aren't any inhaling tubes for children — just one small mask. And we don't have any small needles. I've been advised that Pierre, our commando driver, often goes to Belgrade, so I sent him to the Clinic with a written request to my manager for supplies. He did send me what I asked for, but it took a whole month before I was able to assemble a complete resuscitation kit for infants. Until then, we had to improvise and anesthetize children with Ketalar without intubation whenever it was possible.

As in Knin, there are many children from mixed marriages. The paramedic Saša has a unique problem. He had been working in the OR before I arrived. Then he left, giving as his reason the constant tension, which he found intolerable. He said he was unable to react on time, so he went to the front line as a member of a triage team whose responsibility was to provide immediate emergency care to the wounded. The reason he gave for his resignation didn't make any sense. The front lines are everywhere, so we're all under constant stress. One night, Saša came with a medical team that brought in a wounded soldier. We invited the medical team to stay for a meal of leftovers from dinner. In no time at all, out comes a guitar and a surgeon from Belgrade turns out to be an excellent entertainer. He has dignified, aristocratic features and gentlemanly manners, but he plays passionately. As we started to sing, the bands of fear and tension slackened and life's energy came flowing back. This life is hidden. It occurs behind our closed eyelids. It's the life that we keep to ourselves, that we hide from others. In the semi-darkness, we reveal our true selves and released streams of emotion that cascade across the room. We sang along and applauded the performers from our isolated worlds.

Saša is a good-looking guy. He wears a moustache. He was sitting beside me. A bottle of brandy is being passed around and it's almost empty. Saša is a bit tipsy. He relaxes and starts talking about himself. His mother is a Croat. At the beginning of the war, she left her Serbian husband and two sons to go to the Croatian side. His brother went to Knin right away, where he was later killed. And Saša, profoundly disillusioned, went to the front lines to get himself killed as soon as possible. He's not running away from the OR and its responsibilities — he's running away from himself.

"If only I could erase those bitter memories of my mother!" he complained.

"Why?" I asked him. "I think she would have left even if there had been no war. Your father has a drinking problem. And he abused her. That's what everyone says. Don't attribute everything to nationalism."

But Saša remained embittered. Belief can be a cohesive force that holds the imagination in its grip with one single idea. Nothing will change his mind. Culpability is by far preferable to chaos. I wonder how many lives are likewise coming apart. Saša is only twenty-two but he has already given up hope. He wants to get himself killed. All this will be over someday. But will he be able to forgive his mother and rid himself of guilt for his brother's death before his own death wish comes true?

* * * *

A patient who had suffered a bullet wound to the head was brought in. We opened his skull to release pressure on the brain. The operation lasted four hours, but it wasn't a complete success. The brain had already been damaged by the bullet as well as by severe bleeding. Although the medical staff did their utmost — nothing could be done. The patient died. He was Croatian. It's interesting to note that the United Nations Protection Force (UNPROFOR) showed up immediately afterwards to follow up. There are many wounded soldiers on the Serbian side, but UNPROFOR never inquires about them. I couldn't understand why they were interested only in Croats and Muslims. Soon, it became apparent that these patients' stories made sensational copy for the newspapers. The history of the West's adversarial relationship with Communism colored the favorable coverage in the Western press of the question of Croatian and Bosnian independence, which the press presented as being in the West's best interests. The press is oblivious to the brutal tactics of Croatian separatists inflicted against Serbs during their campaign of ethnic cleansing. The press is also oblivious of the role Middle-Eastern jihadists played in the creation of the Al-Mujahedeen Brigade (306th) of the Bosnian Muslim Army. UNPROFOR soldiers come bearing gifts of cigarettes and chocolate for Croatian and

Muslim patients, but they bring nothing for Serbs. "Next time!" is what they say.

Before coming here, I cherished the hope that the International Community and the United Nations would help us extinguish this blaze. I imagined that they were more interested in justice than expediency. Now I clearly understand that they are not at all interested in the facts. This realization sickens me. I have long been waiting for the moment when representatives of international humanitarian organizations come bearing goodwill and cheer for wounded Serbian soldiers, as well, but "next time" never comes. They are like Saša, under the spell of an *idée fixe*. Their obsession is *independence means justice*. They're sorely mistaken.

White trucks filled with earth rumbled along the streets of Glina. No one knew where UNPROFOR is transporting it. I watch the soldiers' faces, which range from fair red-headed (almost transparent) Nordic men to the blue-black complexions of Nigerians. Some are cleanly shaven, others have long beards. The European Caucasians regard us with insolent scorn. What annoys me the most is that one can easily see that these so-called representatives of the Great Powers are not elite troops, but mercenaries — even sociopaths. I don't have a high opinion of them and no one can convince me that they are actually helping us. Who gave them the right to truck our earth from one place to another? I watch them with growing animosity.

These nightly transports rattle the hospital windows, which causes things to bounce on shelves. The commotion awakens whole town. They are parading their power and instilling fear in the population. The other day, one of the guards in front of the hospital stopped a jeep that was marked *Doctors without Borders*. The passengers wouldn't allow the guards to inspect the vehicle on the grounds that it was against international regulations. Their posturing got them nowhere, because our guards had already opened up the luggage rack where a camera was found with shots of all the important facilities in Glina, along with a few machine guns. They were spies posing as doctors. *Doctors without Borders* was spying on us. These are humanitarians? Peacekeepers? Does the *Doctors without Borders* headquarters know and approve of this? If so, they're a disgrace to the medical profession.

10. Glina

Glina is the second largest town in the province of Banija. Before the war, this charming town had about 6,000 inhabitants. Ironically, the war has caused migration in both directions so now the number of inhabitants remains about the same, but it's composed of different populations. In a majority of cases, people of different nationalities simply exchanged houses. The Croats went to the Croatian part of the territory while the Serbs came here — complete households were left behind by both sides. The property they had been acquiring over the years no longer belonged to them. In fact, there are refugees on both sides who had luckily not ended up on the street; however, there are many others who came with nothing. Most people are living in unfamiliar surroundings. Wherever one turns, everything suddenly belongs to someone else. Uncertainty reigns.

Members of the hospital staff who live in the surrounding villages work, sleep, and have meals at the hospital for several consecutive days. Zora, the Instrument Technician, a woman who has friendly eyes and is always willing to kid around, has to travel 25–30 km from Petrinja. She bicycles, walks, or hitchhikes to the hospital. Once she even hitched a ride on a tank. The only thing that matters to her is arriving on time. Her salary is minimal. She can barely afford a chocolate bar. One lives off the land or from humanitarian aid — although there are many objections as to how these humanitarian aid supplies are being distributed. One lives by working, because work itself is often the best therapy. By working, we socialize. Continual danger doesn't allow us to think about what tomorrow may bring. We live for today because tomorrow may never come.

Some of the population has been killed; others have been wounded. Life is disappearing fast from these regions. (Before my arrival, an anesthetist committed suicide by giving himself a lethal dose of anesthetics. The staff is silent about the tragedy. Depression and apathy are pandemic.) Those who manage to stay alive are fighting for their existence. Life has become simple and instinctive. Here, everyone knows what a smile, a clasp of a hand, a touch means. It's moral support to carry on. It's an expression of delight in every passing moment of life that remains. Personal contact is a part of the struggle to survive. The human cry is: "Please, stand by my side!" Everyone is either seeking security or oblivion. Everyone wants to forget the horrors of everyday life. Humanity, tenderness, and love of life flourish in moments when people are suffering the infliction of the greatest of cruelties.

The hospital in Glina is called "Holy Unmercenary Physicians Cosmas and Damian." It was named after twin brothers who were early Christian physicians and martyrs. The hospital in Knin changed its name to St. Sava, the hospital in Vojnić to ——
——. All the names have changed. Notices on signposts and signboards are now written in Cyrillic. Local self-proclaimed "Patriots" check the signatures of volunteers to see if we signed our names in the Cyrillic or Roman alphabet. In Serbia, we grew up believing that the two alphabets were equal. In Serbia itself, there is more signage in the Roman alphabet than in Cyrillic. All this coercion seems strange and grotesque at a time like this when the world is falling apart. The wealthy residents, whom Serbia thought would be helpful, immediately fled Krajina and went either to Serbia or abroad to protect their interests. Only those who lived in dire poverty remained to defend their homes

and the Serbian character of the region. They have been left to fend for themselves.

But even the poor need security forces, doctors, teachers, and priests to provide the necessary structure for a functioning, sustainable community. Unfortunately, those are the very people who are leaving. Although it may be considered immoral to pay no heed to the wellbeing of the community, those who left were treating the survival of Serbs in Krajina as a mythical illusion. Morality has been pulverized. I am not in a position to judge anyone, but I am sorry that these people will not have doctors to treat their illnesses, teachers to teach their children or priests to guide them spiritually.

Luckily, there are always exceptions. The Director of the Hospital in Glina is Dr. Dario Rajić, a vascular surgeon who has managed to work on his doctoral thesis in spite of the upheavals of war. He is the father of two children, and he is one of those rare intellectuals who stayed in Krajina. Before the war, he worked in Karlovac, whose hospital had been built with voluntary financial contributions from the people of Banija and Kordun, regions where Serbs represented a majority of the population. That hospital met high European standards thanks to its equipment and its staff of specialists. Since most of the hospital staff is now in Glina, I can attest from first-hand experience that they are highly professional.

Dr. Rajić worked for fifteen years in Germany, as well, where he was a highly respected cardio-vascular specialist. His parents had even earned their pensions in Germany. With the money they earned, they built a large, beautiful house near Karlovac. They had an apartment, a large business, and a weekend cottage on the Adriatic coast. They lost everything when the war broke out. Being an excellent physician, Dr. Rajić (whom I came to call Dario) could have chosen to accept an HDZ ID card and thus could have become a member of the Croatian ultranationalist party, in which case all his property and the lives of those dearest to him would have been "spared." But at the core of his being, he was a true Serb, insubordinate and proud. He wouldn't tolerate either pressure or blackmail. He refused an HDZ ID card, so all his property, including his savings accounts in Croatian banks, was confiscated.

He withdrew to Petrova Gora with like-minded people. Dr. Dragojević, a fellow surgeon who was also from Karlovac, joined him. The two of them and an otolaryngologist established the first war hospital in Petrova Gora. At an altitude of 500 meters, beside the War Memorial erected in honor of the victims of Fascism during WWII, yet another war hospital was set up in wooden shacks. Memories of WWII are still palpable in this dense forest of chestnut, oak, and beech trees.

A steep and winding road leads to the hospital. It's difficult to reach after a snowfall. These are nineteenth-century conditions: no electricity, no reliable water supply, and no adequate heating. The physicians still manage to function somehow. Wounded soldiers keep arriving along with civilians whose illnesses require medical treatment. We save lives.

After the first phase of the war ended, the hospital was divided into two separate units, one of which was moved. Dr. Rajić, although he was from the Perna (which is near Kordun), came to Glina where there is an old hospital building. This hospital never had a surgery department, but the structure was adaptable so it was repurposed.

Opposite the improvised ICU and OR, there is a small room where Dr. Dario sleeps. His bed is actually a sofa that was really designed only for sitting. He manages to sleep on it, but since he's a little plump, he can't turn over without risking falling to the floor. Under such conditions, he can never get the full night's sleep he needs to run a hospital, but he doesn't complain. Even though he keeps everything functioning as normally as possible, he still needs a change of scene as well as a chance to relax. Isolation can be just as deadly as a bullet.

Dr. Dragojević went down to Vojnić in Kordun, where he set up a hospital in a former motel. The staff from Petrova Gora, which had until recently worked together, had to be divided between the two hospitals. There aren't enough doctors at either hospital. The specialists often work alone. From time to time, volunteers arrive, but there are never enough of them. The staff is exhausted and their nerves are always on edge. Uncertainty is taking its toll. Many people, who apparently have good intentions, offer to help — but the result is division among the Serbs. We volunteers immediately notice that there is an unspoken division between Banija and Kordun. Kordun is under the patronage of the Church, and it has had a great number of benefactors from abroad. There is more medicine and a greater variety of food. Banija also receives humanitarian aid, but it isn't nearly as generous.

Bishop Nikanor may wear glasses but his short-sightedness in other areas explains why the Church's support does not extend to Banija. In this case, it's his responsibility to remedy the situation.

* * * *

We also find it strange that when humanitarian aid does arrive from abroad, it is practically useless. A huge truck can show up completely full. We all unload it together. Our Director is always with us. After we unpack all the boxes and look at the expiration dates on the medicines, only a rather small box remains that contains valid "best-used-before" dates. Instead of getting a truckload of solution for intravenous feeding, we get half a truckload of catheters for aspiration and medications that are completely inappropriate for wartime use. It's clear now that the "donors" are just clearing out their dispensaries without giving any thought to what we really need. It's sad, but true. We saw it with our own eyes.

* * * *

Even before the war, there was no Operating Room in Glina, but after the arrival of Dr. Rajić, two ORs were constructed with help from the Army. Operating tables were improvised from dentist's chairs. We collected everything that we might need. The ORs that I found when I arrived were relatively decent, but no surgery could be performed in them without sterilization. A surgical procedure may be flawlessly executed but infection can be deadlier than a bullet. Sterilization is carried out in two old Autoclaves, and as Dr. Rajić pointed out, they are expensive, too. The sterilization process is very slow and lasts between four and five hours. Since there are frequent power cuts, our success hinges on the staff in charge of sterilization. There can be no idling because there are always new instruments that have to be sterilized. All of us are extremely conscientious, so there's no malingering. Nothing is left to chance.

Principal Staff Members in the Hospital

Helena

Instrument Technicians are the soul of surgery. This holds true in Glina, too. All of our techs are refugees. They are Serbs who came here from different hospitals on the Croatian side or from abroad to stand by their people in difficult times.

Helena, the Chief Instrument Technician, is a strong and determined woman. Her eagle eye misses nothing, so she keeps our surgical lives under control. When water starts flowing from the taps, plastic barrels, cans, demijohns, fuel cans, and bath tubs are immediately filled. The Autoclaves are filled with water directly from the tap with a hose or from reserves already on hand. It's difficult and burdensome work, but we know that we'll only have as many supplies as we shall have prepared in advance. All the instruments are cleaned immediately. Surgical sets for specific operations are neatly packed in sterile compresses with expiration dates, and they are all organized on shelves. We take the appropriate steps to prevent infections.

Helena comes from Karlovac. She's my age, and she has two children. At the moment, she's living alone because her husband left her for another woman during the war. Now she's a self-supporting single mother as well as a refugee. Helena's entire life — including a new house — remained in Karlovac. She sleeps in the hospital on a free bed with the patients.

Helena doesn't have it easy. She recently found a small rat hole of an apartment. It's completely inappropriate for raising children. She neither has food nor the time to prepare it for them. And where is she going to leave them when she has to go to work? She usually works day and night, anyway. A wood-burning stove was found with some difficulty for her apartment, but it isn't of much help since there is no wood to be found. One cubic meter of firewood cost twenty deutschmarks. Her salary for a month's work is only ten. It's hopeless. Helena has to leave her children with her parents in a village twenty-five kilometers away. They are safe there and they have food. Her parents are farmers who raise cattle and grow vegetables. The produce from the farm feeds all of them, including Helena.

Every other week, if she's free and if there's a lull in the fighting, she goes to the village to visit her children. Transportation is the biggest problem. The local buses stopped running long ago, ever since the gasoline shortage started. She usually goes with a fellow nurse who lives nearby. They hitchhike part of the way, then walk the rest.

This is how she has lived for almost three years. Helena is an effusive woman, full of life, always in high spirits. Where is she going to spend all that energy? What can she hope for? What does the future hold in store for her?

Rada

Rada is the senior of the two Transfusion Technicians. She's also married and has two children. Her husband is fighting on the front. She's often at the hospital for twenty-four hours at a stretch, so her children are either alone or with her at the hospital. She has been living this way for two years, which makes me wonder where this frail woman finds the strength for it all. She's always smiling and ready to crack a joke. We work closely together, so the blood type we need is always ready well before we ever get the wounded patient on the operating table. Whenever she's able to do so, she comes personally to inquire about the operation and estimates of the amount of blood that will be needed. She manages to obtain fresh blood from donors for some young people who were bleeding profusely. She reserves blood drawn from older donors for other older patients. Since all the blood and plasma come from Belgrade, we're able give exact and effective proportions. Whenever we perform major elective surgery, we have to do pre-operative haemodilution. We economize the use of blood by applying techniques that we learned from the finest clinics in the world. Whenever we have a patient whose chest cavity is full of blood, we collect it with Rada's help, and then we later return it via transfusion to the patient during the operation. We can only do this with the complete cooperation of our team. Whenever I ask them if they can do something that will help achieve better results for the patient, they're always ready. I can't help but love them. They're struggling alone; they have nowhere else to go, yet our struggle to save lives unites us.

We often give parties for the hospital staff, to which we also invite members of the Army. Listening to music, singing songs, and dancing are the best way to relieve emotional strain. We dance tirelessly during these parties. The Banija Kolo (a circle dance) is performed here. Couples dance in circles to the changing rhythms of the music. I like this dance, but it wasn't easy to learn. A single oil lamp usually illuminates the room, and an old transistor radio provides the music. And we always have snacks. Sometimes a patient will contribute a few dry sausages. It's nothing extravagant, of course, but everyone takes part in preparing the festivities.

Dr. Rajić agreed to arrange to have the staff take its meals at the hospital. Food is first provided to the patients, then to volunteers, and finally whatever remains goes to the staff. The menu is invariable. It's incredible how potatoes, beans, and rice can be prepared in so many different ways. But I'm particularly annoyed with the rice. One day it's prepared with a touch of diced meat, on another with a splash of diced carrots, and then peas in a continual merry-go-round. I avoid eating it whenever I can, so I often settle for jam and bread, instead. No one complains. I never heard so much as a whisper of discontent.

The bread is delicious. In Glina, the bakery regularly caters to the townspeople and the restaurants that are still open. Bread is delivered directly to the hospital so that staff members who are working the day shift (and who also have no one at home to run errands) can buy it. Unless the hospital staff had its meals here, most of them would go hungry. Humanitarian aid is arriving, but it isn't nearly enough. People are still able to eat thanks to the hard work of Banija's peasants. They raise cattle, and they know how to smoke and dry meat. Since they have neither electricity nor freezers, the peasants resort to tried and true methods of preserving food. The best known specialty is sausages from Banija. They taste like the dry, fragrant sausages that are served with cocktails. There's a plentiful supply of brandy and wine; a delicious juice is made from plums and aromatic *tamjanika* grapes. I tasted it for the first time in my life here. There are no pastries. Eggs are scarce because the farmers don't have anything to feed to the chickens. Occasionally, we have home-made baklava. There are walnuts to be found. We can buy them at the market in the morning on Wednesdays and they're a good substitute chewing gum and cigarettes.

Simo

Whenever Simo, our sole male Instrument Technician (*i.e.*, surgical nurse) goes home, he returns with a bag and draws me aside. He always brings me some home cooking. I'm nevertheless deeply moved and saddened. I wonder why I deserve such attentiveness. He never bothers to explain but only smiles from the corners of his mouth. Simo is twenty-six. Before the war broke out, he worked in Switzerland as an Instrument Technician in a medical center. He was well paid and was living comfortably there. His parents live in Glina, as well as a brother who has small children. His brother was mobilized when the war broke out, so Simo pulled up stakes and returned home. He doesn't say much and he works all the time. He sleeps in the hospital, wherever a free bed can be found.

We volunteers are accorded the privilege of being accommodated permanently in one place, while the others have to look for a place to sleep each night. When there are no free beds, they sleep on benches, chairs or on the floor. I share a room with two local doctors in the Department of Internal Medicine; the men are accommodated in a room with five beds in the Gynecology Department. Towards evening, when we get running water, those of us who aren't on duty stand in line to shower. There's a bathtub in one part of the bathroom which has a shower head that blasts a jet of water in whatever direction it pleases, so we have to run in a circle, scantily dressed, to shower. It's horrible yet comic. Simo gallantly allows all the women go first, after which he takes a cold shower. Simo either goes on foot or hitchhikes whenever he goes home. His village is about fifteen kilometers away. He isn't married and he doesn't have a girlfriend.

"I don't want to have a steady girlfriend, now," he says. "I don't want to be attached to anyone and I don't want anyone to be attached to me. There's a war going on, so we may be cruelly separated. I want to avoid at least that kind of trauma. Besides, where would I find a girlfriend, anyway? Since I'm so busy and have so many responsibilities, who's going to wait around for me? I'm just grateful that I'm still alive."

After my first few days in Glina, I noticed that all the women had their hair nicely done, just as if there were no war going on. The mystery was quickly solved. Simo was also Glina's acting hairdresser. He was handy with a pair of scissors, curlers, and hairbrushes and he kept coming up with the most beautiful, often unusual hairstyles. All the personnel looked so neat and tidy. I felt ashamed of my unruly hair, but he even managed to help me!

Jana

Jana, a Czech woman, is also one of our Instrument Technicians. Our first conversation began when I entered a room where she was reading a book. She spoke softly.

She's a Roman Catholic who married a Serb. She met her husband ten years ago at a seaside resort; then she joined him in Zagreb. She left her house in Bratislava behind and came to live with him. After the war began, they traded their house in Zagreb for one in Glina.

The property exchange process was diverse. Usually the information came by word of mouth. Serbs had been forced to leave their homes in a hurry to flee from areas where there was a Croatian majority in order to come to areas that were populated by Serbs. There, they would meet Croats who lived side by side with Serbs but who had become increasingly aware of the necessity of leaving the territory before war broke out. Thus, it was a blind exchange of real estate. Some people advertised their offers in newspapers. The Internet hasn't been set up here yet.

Jana's husband is serving on the front, so she's alone here working with the rest of us. She could have returned to the Czech Republic. She and her husband have no children. She could have saved her own life, but she didn't want to leave. Love and commitment are powerful forces.

"I can't go now," she says. "I don't need life without love. I don't want to live without truth and loyalty. I'm staying here with my husband and my people. You are my people now. I made the decision to be a Serb."

She was excited to tell me that she had written to Václav Havel, President of the Czech Republic. She was certain that he was interested in knowing the truth, but she received no reply. Jana is forty-six years old. Her beauty is beginning to fade. She isn't at the beginning of her life, but she certainly isn't at the end. She does her best to survive. She raises chickens and makes wine. She misses her beautiful house, which was in one of Zagreb's tony neighborhoods. She grieves over the loss of her music collection. She can't enjoy Bach, Mozart, and Tchaikovsky; her recordings of *Tosca*, *La Traviata* and *The Barber of Seville* were left behind.

But she also feels sorry for the people with whom they had exchanged houses. She thinks they must be forlorn, as well. They left bedroom furniture, along with unused bed linens. For the time being, both families have a place to live. They managed to save their lives. Most people didn't succeed in doing even that much, but this is meager consolation. They still feel cut off and isolated. Starting over is difficult.

"Over there somewhere, where I lived for a whole decade, is my home," she recalled. "It's still there and it's surrounded by roses and fruit trees that my husband and I had planted one by one ... with love ... with love."

Memories come back to her. The Croatian authorities fired her from her hospital job because she was married to a Serb. Sorrow silently embraces us. As I leave, she puts on her glasses slowly and continues reading. Her figure is slightly bent. It's night. She hovers like a shadow against the window. Snow is falling quietly and it's leaving gleaming white accents on the tops of the pines.

11. Mid-winter 1993 — Media Isolation

We maintain contact with the outside world by means of a transistor radio/cassette recorder. We generally listen to the Croatian news instead of Serbian radio-stations because the Croatians manage to jam Serbian programming. There are two local Serbian radio stations: Radio Petrinja and Radio Petrova Gora. Journalists are always in the field, so they often come to the hospital to interview us. We take advantage of these opportunities. In the interviews, we appeal to the population and we address the fighters on the front lines. If there are five of us, we say there are ten. We deliberately lie. When the soldiers hear that doctors are available here, they know that there will be someone to help them if they get wounded. Their families feel more secure, too. They don't worry as much about children and the elderly. They know Serbia is thinking of them, and that they are not alone. The information reaching them over the radio is rain showering parched earth. It helps them endure. Sometimes, when I hear snatches of our own voices on a radio broadcast as they're bringing in the wounded, I realize how information promptly disseminated provides a sense of community and creates peace of mind. We aren't completely isolated. The broadcasts find their way through encirclements and blockades, and then our fears vanish. We know the enemy is listening, too, so we hope that our voices will give them another wrinkle of concern.

Serbia has unfortunately lost the media war. We don't seem to understand the value of information as our enemies do. The Serbian authorities don't realize how valuable it is to broadcast critical information in a timely manner. Here in Glina, there used to be a television studio, but government officials had it destroyed. We assumed this was done to prevent the studio from falling into the hands of Croatian separatists, but present circumstances here have already demonstrated how that decision cost us dearly.

Resentment towards foreign journalists only increases as the war continues. Some of them come completely unprepared — they lack even a basic understanding of the conflict. Flaunting such ignorance, one American journalist asked during the funeral of one unfortunate Serb near Benkovac:

"Why did the Serbs come to Krajina anyway? What were they looking for in Croatia?"

No one understood his question. What exactly was he asking? Didn't he know that Serbs had been living on this territory for at least five hundred years? This land was first under the control of the Austro-Hungarian Empire; then it became part of Yugoslavia — it was never Croatian. Croatia exists now for the first time in modern history. And foreign journalists never took Serbian victims into account.

Defiance and a sense of wounded dignity grew in the mind of Krajina's Serbian population. Consequently, they denied foreign journalists, as well as any foreigners at all, access to Serbian territories. Dignity is deeply ingrained in the Serbian soul. Serbs will not show their pain and certainly will not cry in front of the cameras. This would be seen as putting their misfortunes up for sale to the highest bidder. The Serbian public held the opinion that foreign journalists had arrived with their stories written in advance, regardless of the situation observable in the field. Some of them had clearly been sent by their respective governments to deliberately damage the reputation of the Serbs.

There are always exceptions. There were conscientious journalists who sought to understand the situation and, to tell the truth, they refused to omit significant details about the reality of the situation. Unfortunately, in Krajina separatists dominated among the authorities, and they made sure that even beneficial information never became public. Journalists were publishing reports and photographs that informed the public only of war crimes that Serbs had committed. No news reports were ever broadcast about Serbs who had been attacked in their very homes. No one bothered to report that the Serbs were simply defending themselves; that they were fighting for survival on the very soil they had lived on for centuries.

Resentment against foreign journalists metastasized, as well as against anyone else who carried a notebook. Paranoia is very much alive — but it's not paranoia when they're really trying to kill you. We're physically isolated, but our mental blocks are even worse. There are no local TV or radio stations we can trust to give us reliable news, free of needless ideology, mysticism, and distortion. We would get information daily by word of mouth, and even though it was one sided, we feel safer. These word-of-mouth reports give us direction, either a common goal to achieve or a common enemy to fight.

Media isolation makes everything that really does happen appear foggy — even censored. It's fertile soil for rumors. We're preoccupied with such questions as: *What is the common goal of the Serbian ethnic minority in Croatia? How will it survive? Who will support them, and what can they expect when such support arrives?* The U.S., a symbol of multiculturalism like Yugoslavia, was supposed to give us hope. Why did the U.S. appear to be helping Croatia in its policy to make the country mono-ethnic? And why was the International Community ignoring the rights of Serbs who have lived here for five centuries? Did the International Community actually want ethnically homogenous countries? Croats wanted to expel the Krajina Serbs, convert them to Roman Catholicism, or simply kill them. In the eyes of Krajina Serbs, Serbia was just a faraway country to which they were not particularly connected. Serbia may be the same nation genetically, but sociologically and epigenetically, it's not the same nation anymore. No one in Serbia even knows about the problems these people in Krajina are facing, so they have no empathy for them. Besides, Serbia is suffering from a severe economic crisis caused by sanctions, so its people are most concerned with the price of groceries, bread, and milk.

There are many paradoxes. A free, reliable, local media could offer some answers. We would have had an easier time understanding what others are thinking and why. But, as things stand, we're completely cut off from the outside world. We're suspended "between the earth and the sky," as the saying goes.

* * * *

A colleague of mine ended up giving a passage from my diary to a journalist. We were hoping that a story about this tragedy would motivate more volunteers to come and help, but we got no response. Then we waited, but still no one came.

We do our best under the circumstances. Whenever we are faced with a problem that either exceeds our competence or the limits of our facilities, we send the patient to Banja Luka or to Belgrade. I call all the institutions that can be of some help. When I don't know what to do with a patient, I get helpful advice from the doctors in Banja Luka. I often speak to Dr. Bilbija on the phone. As a senior surgeon, he gives me medical advice, but he also helps me facilitate the in-take of patients who have to be sent to Banja Luka for further treatment.

His answer is always reassuringly the same: "Send them!"

To be admitted to a hospital in Belgrade, the patient needs a form, a paper certificate, filled out by a doctor, but Krajina has no infrastructure to support health insurance. That causes problems, so I always emphasize to colleagues in Belgrade or Banja Luka whom I'm asking for help:

"They don't have a doctor's form and they don't have any money!"

"They don't need any of that stuff. Just tell them to mention your name..." is the answer.

My colleagues in Belgrade keep their promises. It's easier for us as well as for the patients. Many doctors support us this way; it isn't necessary for them to come here. Honorable people will always find others who are willing to help. It remains to be seen, however, who is going to win the war. Yet I remain certain that civilization will to prevail over barbarity.

In an area of 250,000 inhabitants, there are only two medical facilities where Serbs can get treatment. One is in Vojnić where a hostel serves as an improvised hospital, and the other is here in Glina where the Health Center has also been converted into a hospital. One nurse-anesthetist from Serbia came to work in Vojnić along with a volunteer, while I was left completely alone in Glina, where I remained the only volunteer from Serbia. This is the sorry state of available medical resources in Krajina, which has no centralized coordination. Krajina has been all but forgotten except by a few volunteers from Serbia. Anesthetists perform uncomplicated procedures on patients in Vojnić, while patients with more complicated cases have to be transported to Glina — that is, unless the patient's condition and the attendant safety concerns make the transfer impossible. Glina is 60 km away from Vojnić, and the roads are not always secure. Vehicles are regularly blown up by land mines that were planted along the roads. Nothing is safe.

The nurse-anesthetist in Vojnić is a highly skilled retired military officer. He can operate at the same level as the doctors. I would give anything for a chance to work with him again. Too much responsibility is overwhelming me. I'm not experienced enough to be tackling so much — but that's my problem. I have absolutely no one to whom I can complain. When patients arrive from Vojnić, they come to me not because I'm a better anesthesiologist but because I have a better knowledge of Intensive Care Unit procedures and because I have a better post-operative care team. Sometimes, no other anesthesiologist is present in the hospital, so the patient has no choice but to see me.

Everything is chaotic. Military and civilian agencies are in charge, but they have a poor level of cooperation. There's always a problem about who's going to be in charge and who's going to have the final say. Criminal activity and political corruption are ubiquitous. Criminal organizations arose in the absence of clear law enforcement structures. Sometimes these criminal organizations seize power indirectly by sowing fear and creating an atmosphere of greater insecurity. The legal mechanism is ponderously slow, while criminals are extremely effective in speedily executing their plans. The message is clear: the people, having no legal recourse, must obey the criminals.

There's no money, but drugs are widely available. We have no way of knowing at the hospital what the makeup is of the population we were treating. We can never fully analyze our data because everything changes daily. People keep leaving and new people keep arriving through the revolving door. We're unable to estimate the amount of supplies we need. To make matters worse, there's no way of obtaining either the supplies or the medical personnel we need.

12. Trauma Takes a Psychological Toll

The people of Krajina have been living in isolation for a long time. Constant tension and a long history of stressful circumstances have forced them to live in their own world. They don't always have the strength to face the real world. But the tension is growing uncontrollably. Many of us are boiling over with anger just as steam rattles the sputtering lid of a pot. Many of us have no idea why we're behaving as we do.

To make matters worse, it's difficult under wartime conditions to determine which of our colleagues are certifiably insane and which ones are not. Even so, it's true that there are some people whose behavior is genuinely deranged. These people are, of course, difficult to work with and they have problems getting along with others. Sometimes, it's not necessary to be insane. It's enough to have been traumatized to harm a patient and cause problems for the whole team.

Among the volunteers, there are many medical professionals who do their job capably. But there are a few who have violent tempers or who are psychopaths who have already been barred from working in Serbia. And, of course, there are the idealists who have the skills but the wartime realities are more than they can handle. Gathered in one place, isolated by mountains and roads made impassable by huge snowfalls, we are left to our own devices. We haven't chosen each other; we don't even like one another; and sometimes we feel such tension that we're on the verge of exploding.

Dr. Bojan from Rijeka (in northern Croatia), who is a surgeon and who was also an outstanding student — one of the best at the Zagreb University School of Medicine — is one of those time bombs ready to explode. He possesses a great deal of theoretical knowledge, but his mind is detail-oriented so he's unable to grasp the big picture. He lacks confidence when he has to make a decision. Since we're understaffed, it follows that there is never time for lengthy discussions. It's difficult to figure out what happened to him. Only some nightmare scenario in his life could have toppled him from the heights of accomplishment and then hurled him brutally to the ground.

He was an extraordinary student, but after graduation, just as he began serving his internship as a surgeon, the war broke out. He's a Serb married to a Croat. This young, ambitious man in love saw his world smashed to pieces. His hopes lie hidden behind a thick and impenetrable patriotic fog. He's a good person, somewhat romantic but dedicated to his work. He's not interested in politics. He's only interested in science and his wife. Now, however, his life with his wife and new child is in jeopardy. He decided to get her away from the war zone, so he exchanged their house in Croatia for one in Vojvodina in Serbia. The exchange wasn't a fair trade because they gave up a comfortable house for a shanty. But it was absolutely necessary for him to find a place where his wife and child could be safe. With a heavy heart, he left them in Serbia; then he returned to his birthplace to serve as a doctor.

Working conditions were terrible. There was no hospital, no other surgeons, and no anesthesiologist. He worked with medical personnel from nursing schools. The war was spreading and casualties were mounting at an alarming rate. One day, he sent a seriously wounded soldier to Knin in an ambulance with two nurses. A Croatian grenade hit the ambulance. One nurse and the wounded soldier were killed. The other nurse, Jadranka, was in a coma for a month. She survived but is permanently disabled. That grenade not only hit the medical corps transporting the wounded, but it also hit our surgeon and scarred him for life. Unbearable responsibility had fallen on his inexperienced shoulders while he was already staggering from the blows of other losses.

Dr. Bojan developed meningitis. Even people with stronger constitutions than his have had nervous breakdowns that weakened their immune systems and allowed bacteria to attack. Dr.

Bojan was paralyzed by the disease so he had to be transported by helicopter to the VMA Military Hospital in Belgrade. He was unconscious for a long time. He was unable to give either his own or his family's address — not to mention his surname. No one was able to locate his wife who, meanwhile, was moving from one place to another in Serbia; and no one was able to locate his family, which was still in Krajina. He was in the hospital for six months. No one visited him during that time.

A lot of patients have been admitted to the VMA Hospital in Belgrade, and new ones keep arriving all the time. The medical staff that works in this multi-ethnic hospital is constantly changing. Staff members who originally came from areas that are now newly declared countries often decide to move back home, so their positions are taken by Serbs who have been expelled from those very same new countries. It's impossible to establish continuity in patient care and treatment, so we're unable to follow individual patients because staff members keep coming and going through a revolving door. I did not have an opportunity to visit Dr. Bojan at the VMA. Smederevo is 46 km from Belgrade. Moreover, I had to stop traveling back and forth between Belgrade and Smederevo because the economy was collapsing. We all had to choose between two liters of vegetable oil (which covered the monthly needs of a family) and a one-way bus ticket to Belgrade. No matter how noble people wanted to be, the economic conditions acted as a limiting factor. The question was always: *Should the family or someone else take priority?* Act of kindness are rare.

Dr. Bojan struggled to get well. After a long and difficult convalescence, he returned to work, but he hadn't completely recovered. His parents were in Krajina, but his wife and child were still in Serbia. He was a patriot in the simplest sense of the word: loyal to his native soil. Many disappeared long ago from their native land and left their previous lives behind. He, nevertheless, felt obliged to return and help.

To everyone's regret, he was incapable of discharging his responsibilities. When a surgeon does not work for a long period of time, he loses his touch. And when he cannot be made aware of his shortcomings, it hurts not only the patient but the entire team. This was the dilemma we faced. At first, we felt sorry for him and we tried to make allowances. We understood that he was unhappy, confused, and sick. But simply understanding his misfortune isn't going to help our morale. In the evenings, before the TV news begins, we sit together and watch — or rather listen because the image on the monitor is frequently distorted. We're exhausted and under stress due to long periods of isolation. Either we're silent or we're quietly joking among ourselves in order to reduce tensions. When one staff member becomes anxious, then others become anxious and uncooperative in a chain reaction. We're all afraid of this happening, so we stopped speaking. We no longer have the luxury of griping and gossiping to each other as people normally do. Any expression of fear or uncertainty is unacceptable.

Whenever Dr. Bojan appears, it feels like room was going to explode. He has forebodings of a conspiracy against him and he talks endlessly about it. We remain silent as he, sniffling and coughing lightly, paces the whole evening from the window to the front door and back again. His clogs magnify the noisy rhythm of his neurotic footsteps. He no longer senses the effect he's creating on his environment.

"Well, my friends, you don't know what trouble is," he mutters. "You don't give a fuck — excuse me for swearing. I didn't mean to be indecent. I'm a good man, really ... you just don't give a damn about all that I went through."

We've listened to this story at least ten times already. Each one of us has some difficulty that we either talk about or don't, which depends on the level of distress and the character of the person in question. No one's life is problem-free. On the contrary, only those who have suffered can understand and help others who are suffering. Dr. Bojan can't accept this, so his obsession with his personal problems only intensifies his loneliness. We've all lost patience with him, so we avoid him.

One day, the hospital director calls me in and says: "Doctor Mitić, if anyone understands people, you do. Help him!"

"Dr. Dario, he's a *very* difficult person. You also understand that he's almost incompetent as a surgeon, don't you?"

"O, I don't know. You are going to leave one day, but we're going to have to stay. He belongs to our team and we need him here. Besides, what do you know about surgery, anyway? You're an anesthesiologist," he added with a smile. "But please, take him for a walk. Talk to him. You have a way with people. Be a sport."

So we start taking walks in the bitterly cold winter rain, and we continue them into the first sunny days of spring. We get to know each other better. At first our pace was brisk, but later it slowed down. He shows me wallet photos of his wife and child. His wife is a raven-haired woman with striking features; his child is fragile with pretty eyes.

"Your wife is a very beautiful woman! Now I see why you're worrying about her," I say, trying to joke with him.

"O, yes, she is beautiful. Do you really think that she's beautiful?" he adds suspiciously.

"O, my God, yes. Anyone can see that she's beautiful," I continue, now quite serious.

"She's a devil, a real devil. We really got along so well together. She took care of me, cooked, did the laundry, and waited for me while I was doing my internship. It was wonderful until the war began. Now when I go home she treats me with contempt. Please, don't tell anyone. They'll only laugh at me. I've nowhere to go to get peace of mind."

"Maybe you should find someone else. Get a divorce. Let her go back to Croatia and stay with her parents," I suggest.

"I couldn't do that. She's a good person. But the war has changed her. Our neighbors in Serbia are good to her, but she is a young woman and she's alone. On the one hand, I can't find a job in Serbia; on the other hand, I can't leave my people."

"Why don't you bring her here? We can ask Dr. Dario to find an apartment for you."

"I would like that. We must be together, come what may."

After we returned from this walk, I reported everything to Dr. Dario. He did his best to find an apartment, which, to tell the truth, was empty. We had to provide all the essentials. Then we waited for his wife to come. And after she did arrive, it became clear within few weeks that she wasn't going to endure the pressure of life in the front lines. She left the child with her husband and went home to her family in Croatia. Dr. Bojan, who was already at his wits end, was again swept away by a gale of misery and helplessness. He lost interest in his house as well as in his territory. Everything is meaningless without love.

A large number of marriages are falling apart in the same way. Insanity first destroys emotions, then it breaks hearts.

After a while, I heard from my colleagues in Banija that Dr. Bojan had found a new wife, remarried, and had another daughter, which changed his life completely. Dr. Dario was right. What he needed was understanding and help. But good advice can only be of help if it's given by the right person.

Dr. Dario then asked me to extend my stay yet again, because they would have been left without an anesthesiologist, and there was only a slim chance of getting a new one while the fighting was still going on. But I was longing to see my children, as well. I felt the pangs of conscience for not being with them. Even so, the thought of leaving the hospital without an anesthesiologist paralyzed me. Once again I was on the horns of a dilemma.

I decided to stay.

Dr. Dario comforts me: "There is nothing wrong with you being here. Your children are well. If necessary, we'll provide money to make sure that they are looked after."

"No, that won't be necessary," I reply. "My children are doing well. They have everything they need, except their mother. I'm just a little worn out. I've been living in close quarters for a long time with the same people and problems."

Dr. Dario nods in agreement. He understands.

13. The JNA Commander in Glina – Colonel Marko Vrcelj

Tonight, an entire battalion of the Serbian Army of Krajina[17] from Banija and Kordun is mobilizing to aid in the defense of Lika and Dalmatia. The groups rotate every fifteen days. Many of the first to leave are now returning in coffins. Everyone at the hospital is listening to reports from the Dalmatian battlefield, where the husbands and brothers of many our nurses are serving. All of us are keeping a fearful count of the days remaining until their return. When the last group from Dalmatia arrives, Glina reverberates with shouts of joy and the sound of celebratory gunfire. It's difficult for those who are leaving, and not in the least for Glina's commander, Colonel Marko Vrcelj.

Colonel Vrcelj spent most of his adult life as a soldier in Slovenia. He left behind everything he had there. Long before the war, he sensed trouble brewing, so he warned the JNA leadership

---

17. *the Serbian Army of Krajina* (Serbian: Српска Војска Крајине, *Srpska Vojska Krajine*) was officially formed on March 19, 1992.

that something strange was going on in Slovenia. Yugoslavia was not loved by everyone. But the leadership ignored his warnings. Now we're all being punished for their blindness. The Colonel paid a heavy price for their mistakes. He was denounced, and ousted from his post just as many other honest Yugoslav officers were. His son, Vladimir, a boy of fifteen, is in the battlefield with his father (which is unheard of!) where he shares his father's as well as his people's destiny. Until recently, Vladimir had been in the village of Dragotina, lodging in the house of one of the other fighters, while the Colonel slept in his office on an iron camp bed. They saw each other only occasionally. Now they have an apartment, but they still didn't see one another often. A soldier's duties don't allow much free time.

Many mothers here are wearing black scarves of mourning. With Dr. Privanović, we gather the mangled bodies of the dead with our own hands and place them in black plastic body bags. We do that in order spare the fighters the pain of reliving the scenes of carnage. For days after that, I am in shock. I can't even open my mouth. My colleagues force me to drink water sweetened with sugar. My brain is whirling. I keep seeing the body bags for a long time afterwards. I clasp their sad mothers' hands after I offer them condolences, which only magnifies my outrage and defiance. World War II must not be repeated.

The atmosphere is tense. Colonel Vrcelj has beautiful blue eyes shadowed by sorrow.

"Evil times are coming," he says. "Strange things are happening in Russia. Tomorrow is the Assembly in Beli Manastir. Who knows? One can only imagine what will happen next. Dangerously divergent points of view can mean our defeat. It will be very difficult to look at Serbs who score a victory at the expense of their own people. It will be difficult to see that and yet to love them at the same time."

And he does love them. Otherwise, he wouldn't be able to endure all the humiliation and harassment to which he has been subjected since his arrival. Once he was appointed Commander, order was established in Glina. It's authentic military rule that imposes clear responsibilities on the residents. Many of them don't like it. Those who go "fishing in muddy waters" and who want to profit from the chaos are against the Colonel. He's too strict for them. Thieves prefer chaos; they don't like discipline and responsibility.

The number of mobilized soldiers rose to the absolute limit. Then the economy began to revive after a slowdown in the fighting. Conscription for the Army is carried out in the best possible way. The Colonel stimulates the private sector by proving himself to be a man the people can trust, because he has restored a higher degree of security and self-respect to the people. He has survived several assassination attempts but he never flinches from doing his duty — he isn't afraid of death, but he swears that while he is the commander, no Serb is going to get killed by another Serb. (And the Colonel did survive. After he left, however, criminals killed the commander who replaced him.)

In his earnest desire to establish a legitimate state, the Colonel has submitted about a hundred and fifty criminal charges to the local court, but not one single case is being brought to trial. Thus, the judicial system is sabotaging everything that the Army is trying to do for the community. There is a vast chasm between the civilian and military authorities. This discord is aided and abetted by outside factors, and no one can tell right from wrong in such a tense atmosphere. This is why the firm hand of Colonel Vrcelj established a desperately needed sense of security. And he works hard to be a military figure they can rely on. He solves problems by taking systematic measures. Passivity has harmful effects. People think it's sufficient that they themselves do no harm, but it's not enough. They have to prevent others from committing criminal acts. In such critical moments, everyone has to act together to fight the encroaching evil, and it's just as important to join forces to oppose criminality in our own ranks. Nevertheless, it's difficult to decide which of our own people to support when the chain of command is so unstable. There's no clear plan as to where Krajina belongs or where it's going. There's a big difference between those who are respected by the majority of the people in Krajina and those who have been imposed on them by authorities in Serbia.

Commander Vrcelj and I finally met at the celebration of Women's Day on March 8 at the hospital. Doctor Martinović had been trying to introduce us for a long time, but I skillfully managed to avoid it. I heard from the nurses, as well as from the director of the hospital, that the Commander was an obdurate, rough, narrow-minded, and strict soldier. There was no kidding around with him. He strictly enforces the rules, and he confiscates weapons from civilians in Glina. In other parts of Krajina, there are large quantities of weapons in the hands of civilians, but here, the Colonel confiscated them and issued permits only to those whom he allowed to carry weapons. That was why some doctors went to Prijedor to get guns, because it wasn't easy to purchase one in Glina. I don't want a weapon. I saw a gun dealer put a pistol to a customer's throat because the customer was unhappy about the price. It's important to avoid such scenes.

We used to celebrate Women's Day in the former Yugoslavia, and nothing could have prevented us from observing it now. Of course, women's equality is an important legacy from the Second World War. But here, the most important thing is to create a social life for ourselves. We need some fun and entertainment to forget the war, at least for a little while.

Since we have no entertainment budget, Dr. Dario bought a piglet with his own money. And I went into the woods to collect green pine branches to decorate the hall. I was trembling with fear all the while. Representatives of the Army from Glina, as well as from Kordun, were invited to the celebration. I already heard many good things about the Commander from Kordun, Colonel Bulat, so I was glad to meet him. But I didn't want to meet the Commander from Glina, even though he had promised to come. The celebration was well under way and the guys had started to play music. Laughter and high spirits reigned just as if there were no war going on. Colonel Bulat had not yet arrived.

I'm a little sad and worn out. There's a patient in the improvised ICU who's not doing well and I don't know how to help him. The surgeon who could have operated on him is on a trip, so I'm stymied when it comes to considerations for his continued medical treatment. While I'm weighing all the possibilities, a crowd gathers around me. Dr. Dario greets me with teasing.

"What's the matter, Doctor, aren't there any fine gentlemen here to put a smile on your face?"

I don't pay attention to his poor attempt at humor.

"No, there aren't any real men here, Comrade Dario," I say, replying arrogantly in order to discourage him. "That's why this war has lasted so long."

After I make this sharp rebuke, I feel a hand on my shoulder. I have to turn around. In front of me is a man whom I don't know. He has the most beautiful smile in the world.

"Doctor, I'd like to ask you for a dance. I don't know whether I'm a good dancer or not … because that always depends on the woman. She has to inspire her partner to dance well. But it would be my pleasure!"

With a sure hand, he almost lifts me off the floor and I, surprised and bemused by his initiative, can't help but dance with him. His hands are warm; his touch pleasant. The music relaxes me; I follow him. He dances elegantly in his combat boots. Our conversation also starts flowing freely. I begin laughing without being aware of it. One dance follows another, and it never occurs to me to change partners. As we dance, he whirls me around quickly here and there and my temperament starts getting the better of me. I break into a smile and I say in my most innocent voice:

"Goodness, you're so pleasant and agile! I didn't know that officers could actually dance. You're nothing like the Glina Commander. People say he's ramrod straight and cold-hearted. You're so warm. It's not typical of officers."

He laughs quietly. His enigmatic smile returns, which makes his face exceptionally handsome as he twirls me. It really has been a long time since I felt such elation and warmth of heart.

Suddenly, the Intensive Care nurse comes into the hall and interrupts the dance. I have to go. My patient has taken a turn for the worse, so something has to be done. I thank the officer for the dance and I run after the nurse.

I stay in the ICU for more than an hour, and then on my way back up the stairs of the Administration Building, where the celebration is taking place, I find my charming, handsome dance partner. Behind him, I see other soldiers leaving the building. It's just the right moment to thank him once again for a pleasant evening.

Just then, Dr. Martinović comes by and says: "I'm really glad that you two have finally met. It's about time!"

"Whom have I met?" I ask, cautiously expecting a disagreeable answer.

"Why this is Commander Vrcelj, Doctor. Didn't he introduce himself to you?" asks Dr. Martinović, and he continues rather pompously. "This is our renowned Marko Vrcelj, Commander of Glina."

A chill comes over me. I'm ashamed of everything I had said while we were dancing. I was talking about *him*. But I can't do anything about it now. That was what I had heard about him, which was someone else's opinion. At least I was honest. But I shouldn't have been talking about someone I didn't know at all.

I raise my head, blushing scarlet, and I accept his hand, which he has extended.

"Well, it was a great pleasure to meet you Colonel, and thank you for the lovely dance. Unfortunately, I have shown myself in my true light. Now you know that I like to talk."

"Thank you, Doctor. I personally don't have problems with either women's voices or honest judgments. I have more problems with those who don't say anything or who are just plain dishonest. I have to go now, but we'll be seeing more of each other soon, I'm sure!"

My heart leapt. Despite all the unpleasant stories about him, I discovered that he was quite a fine man.

I didn't have to wait long to see him again. He soon came to the hospital and asked the Director what the Army could do to help. He had heard that the hospital needed many things. Perhaps the Army could be of help in matters of mutual interest.

I met him in the corridor where the Director was smiling, and he said: "Doctor, we couldn't force Colonel Vrcelj to come to the hospital even under the threat of arms, but now he's showing up voluntarily, and he's even going to help us. Do you, by any chance, have anything to do with this?"

"Goodness gracious, no, Dr. Dario. How could I? The Commander is fair and just, and he's ready to help. That must be the reason why he came."

The Commander and I are smiling at each other and the light coming from our eyes is saying much more than a simple hello.

I think I really like this man!

I complain that we don't have enough blankets and that we're freezing. We understand that the Army had plenty of blankets, but we did not know how to go about getting them. Dr. Dario says that he's going to send me to Kordun to scrounge up some blankets from his friend, Colonel Bulat. It's starting to look like I have a way with officers.

After I managed to soften up Vrcelj, Bulat, who's a warmer personality to begin with, decided that he was going to give us everything we needed.

Now I'm offended, so I retort sharply to Dr. Dario:

"If you think I'm going to prostitute myself for a pile of blankets, you can forget about it!"

"No, Doctor, you don't have to prostitute yourself. Clever women are able to solve their problems with a smile and a display of kindness. Beautiful women like you pull it off even more gracefully. Bulat is a real gentleman. All you have to do is show him some kindness and ask him nicely. I'm sure he'll give you everything that he possibly can. I'll talk to him. Meanwhile, get ready to hit the road. Those blankets aren't going to come here on their own. You've got to go and get 'em."

This rational, reticent man made me feel ashamed of myself. He's right. Tension and stress have given me a bitter edginess. I've lost touch with my femininity. I didn't realize that I had changed so much. I don't know if I'm ever again going to be the woman I used to be before I came here.

14. Kordun

Dr. Dario tells me that he heard from reliable sources in Serbia that my husband Miroslav had allegedly had an affair with his best friend's ex-wife. His jealous ex-friend then fired a few shots at him and now rumors about the affair are making the rounds in Smederevo. It even merited a newspaper headline:

DIRECTOR OF SMEDEREVO PUBLIC REVENUE OFFICE
CAUGHT PANTS DOWN WITH HIS HONEY POT
WHILE HIS WIFE IS ON THE FRONT LINES IN KRAJINA

The article reports that Miroslav ran out into the street dressed only in his underwear while his ex-friend was chasing him with a gun. It sounds tragi-comic. I don't know whether to laugh or to cry. I try to imagine chubby Miroslav running a zig-zag pattern to dodge bullets. I don't even know if there's a grain of truth to the story. Even so, one thing is quite clear. Miroslav has indeed initiated divorce proceedings. He promised that he was going to protect me and my children from those who were threatening to kill him. One sure-fire way of getting a divorce is to have an affair. This is no longer a putative agreement or a plausible plan. It's happening right now. It's tearing me apart. An invisible but palpable breach is opening between us.

This is another turning point in my life: one more separation. And it saddens me. There's something ominous in the wind but I can't help Miroslav. My sorrow can't be any deeper than it already is. I realize that I haven't hit rock bottom yet. I just can't admit defeat. What's in store for me now when I return to Serbia? How are my children going to react to all this? It grieves me to be apart from them.

* * * *

We weren't able to meet our colleagues from Krnjak on our first trip to Kordun, but a week later we were invited to a party that was being held in a restaurant on the road to Kordun. The volunteers from Krnjak had also been invited. And Milo Paspalj, the President of the Parliament of the Republic of Krajina, arrived. I remember him from Knin, when he was stumbling over words as he was reading the constitution of this unfortunate Republic that no one recognizes. He arrived in Glina wearing a silk shirt and trousers. Massive gold chains adorned his neck and wrists. It's terribly thoughtless of him to dress so tastelessly before starving people. Dr. Dario receives him in his capacity as Hospital Director with all the pomp and circumstance that Paspalj's office demands. Dr. Dario asks me to entertain our "President." People who hold political office are entitled to be treated with respect. I greet Paspalj, who is leaning back in his chair with his legs stretched out like a drunken movie cowboy. I have to stoop to shake his hand. All this is a little strange and slightly offensive. I'm obviously not the right person to entertain this idle President of a nonexistent country whose unfortunate residents I'm treating.

"Dr. Dario, I'm sorry but I'm not a night club hostess," I say, whispering loud enough so Paspalj can hear me. Dr. Dario stares daggers at me. I know he's deeply annoyed by my behavior.

"No one would pay you to entertain anyone, anyway, with that venomous tongue of yours!" he shouts.

My face is contorted by anger as I run off to my room. All of you be damned! I thought.

A little later, we all arrive at the restaurant where the celebration is being held. It's going to be a special luncheon with live music. Our colleagues from Kordun have already arrived. Roast lamb is being served, which is a great delicacy compared to our usual fare. Dr. Elmez jokes that even the neighborhood dogs don't like us volunteers.

"Why?" I ask him, a little puzzled.

"Because we gnaw at bones until there's nothing left for them! We go through food just as locusts cut through grass!"

This sets off a round of laughter.

Marko Vrcelj, the Glina Commander, enters the hall with his entourage. He calmly goes to the other side of the room and settles into a chair. I'm glad to see him again. He nods his head in a friendly manner and I can see a smile on his face that wrinkles the corners of his eyes. I'm glad he's here. It makes me feel more comfortable. Then Milo Paspalj enters. Everyone runs to greet him. Dr. Dario introduces him to the doctors, including our colleagues from Kordun. He extends his hand to the doctors, but he skips me and proceeds to extend his hand to Dr. Elmez, who's sitting at my side. Dr. Elmez did not reciprocate, but says coldly that if President Paspalj doesn't want to shake hands with me, then he has no reason to shake hands with him. Paspalj is nonplussed, but he ignores me. He proceeds to extend his hand to the next person, who also refuses to shake his hand.

"If Dr. Sarah is not good enough for you, then we aren't either. So the best thing for us to do would be to pack up and leave."

Paspalj is startled, but he smooths things over with a smile and says: "Here in Banija we shake hands only with men — and not with women. But since you insist, I'll shake her hand, too!"

I'm boiling with anger and humiliation. I'm unable to compose myself. When he tries to shake hands with me again, I rise from the table and say, spitting out the words: "Back in Serbia, we only shake hands with human beings. That's why I can't shake your hand!"

I head straight for the door. Unpleasant silence fills the restaurant, interrupted only by the sound of a chair creaking nervously. Someone suddenly turns on loud music. A nurse runs to Dr. Paspalj and pulls him into a dance which defuses the situation. Someone grabs my hand before I reached the door and draws back. It's Commander Marko.

"Come on, let's dance! I wouldn't miss this dance for anything in the world," he says, cajoling me. "It'll help you relax."

I draw close to him and we start dancing. I'm about to cry on his shoulder. He presses me even closer. I don't resist. I need so much to be held.

We're suddenly jarred by loud, reverberating explosions that light up the sky outside. One explosion follows another in a continual barrage. We stay calm, yet we're frightened. Commander Marko leaves my side and runs out first. I quickly find myself following him. The sky is reddening from the distant explosions. It turns out that the Army is clearing mines that the enemy has planted in the fields, mines intended to kill unknowing farmers during the sowing season. It's better to intentionally detonate them now rather than to lose lives later.

We stand gazing at the spectacle. The others don't stay outside long. Once they're convinced that they aren't in any danger, they pick up partying where they left off. I'm cold because I'm just wearing a thin dress. The wind is picking up. I start shivering. Marko gently draws me close and warms me with his body. In an instant his lips are on mine and his hands are in my bra. This man knows what he wants and how to get it. I lean into him and return his kiss. Then reality comes roaring back in the form of an ambulance I see approaching out of the corner of my eye. In the time it takes to smooth my dress, the ambulance comes to a stop in front of us and cuts short our brief escapade. The driver opens the door and shouts: "Hop in, Doc! The surgeon's waiting for you."

Back to work, back to war. Here, neither I nor the Commander have private lives. That's why these spontaneously stolen moments are so precious. They are the sunshine on which my life depends. I hop gingerly into the ambulance as a gust of wind lifts my skirt. The Commander puts his hand gently on my bare knees and caresses them. I look him tenderly in the eyes, and then I close the door slowly. The ambulance has already started pulling away. Our moment has ended.

At the hospital, I rush to change my clothes and dash into the OR. Hours later, very late at night, I'm still in the OR ventilating a patient who is still under anesthesia. Dara comes into the room and tells me that I have a visitor. A visitor? I think. In the middle of the night? I hand her the balloon and go out. There, in our break room, sits Commander Marko, waiting for me with the most beautiful smile in the world on his face. The charming rogue says he has nowhere to sleep tonight because his son locked him out. So, can he spend the night here? I'm about to tell him that I have no room of my own when *he* produces the key to my room, and says: "Dara's sleeping somewhere else tonight. I'll meet you upstairs."

I laugh out loud. The scoundrel! This guy is persistent and he knows how to organize things.

A little later, the operation is over and I move the patient to the ICU. Dara is going to take over and attend to him. I wash up and put on my sexiest under things. It's been a long time. My marriage to Miroslav didn't include sex. I didn't even dare think about it. I'm actually trembling out of a profound need to be held, to be given a little sense of security. I've been in this wind-swept hold-out region where I've been giving and giving, yet where I've been frightened for such a long time.

I enter the room and begin to undress. I don't take off my underthings because I think I look sexier that way. Outside the moon is shining through the half-open window pane, where I see my reflection dissolving into the moonlight.

Marko turns abruptly and says: "Why didn't you take those things off?"

He speaks with a sense of urgency. It's high time I forgot about romance, lingerie, and bedroom fantasies! I slip under the covers. His firm but warm soldier's body awaits me. I don't resist. He covers me with kisses. His hands touch me, caress me just as a musician fingers an instrument. I had almost forgotten how it felt!

15. Love and War

Morning erupts in the bedroom with the clamor of soldier's boots, which startles me from my light sleep. Marko posted a guard in front of the door with instructions to wake him before roll call. The soldier is now obediently carrying out the order. Marko dons his uniform in a flash. He lovingly pulls the covers over me, then plants a kiss on my forehead.

"See you soon!" he says tenderly. "You and I are going to be seeing a lot more of each other."

I take a deep breath and try to hold on to him just a little longer. I lock my lips to his. I'm not going to let him get away that easily.

My flesh longs for his touch. I still feel his kisses fluttering on the nape of my neck. A sweet chill runs down my thighs and tightens my back. Tenderness flows from his hands. My breasts swell. Two desires, one a bow and the other an arrow, unite to hit the target. I feel a *frisson* of resonant, sweet cool air. Our lips find their way in the dark, and they want to give as good as they get.

O, God, please make this last! My weary head lays on his warm, firm and manly chest. His powerful biceps cushion me. My lips search for the hollow of his throat. We say that's where the soul lives. That's where a tender kiss should go. Then we hold each other tightly in an embrace. Could there be some personal feeling in all this? Are our bodies simply rejoicing because of genuine desire or because of the need to discharge the pent up emotions that result from dealing with chaos?

And then he was gone.

That was the first of many such mornings when I saw him off from my room. We had nowhere else to go. Even so, I wanted more.

"Don't cry," he'd say. "Your smile will follow me into battle. And so will your optimism, your love for life, your love for everything beautiful. It's fine that you're more in love with love than you are with me. You're acting as if each time we meet is going to be our last."

I hear the echo of his boots, which take him to new uncertainties. The war, a black curtain draping us, can't suppress the radiance of love. The uncertainty of when our next rendezvous will take place only makes my longing for him more keenly felt. I hold his kisses to my lips with my fingertips to keep them from vanishing. The bed holds his scent. This woman is going to wait for her soldier to come back — but I end up dreading the possibility that each arriving ambulance might be carrying his maimed body.

Marko comes to visit me whenever it's possible. Sometimes he takes me for a ride around Glina to show me the sights. He loves this country. He'd sometimes crumble a clod of earth in his hand, letting it sift slowly through his fingers, and he'd say: "Look how rich this soil is! When the war's over, it'll yield wheat and feed livestock as well as people. Everything will return to the soil again. It's a natural process. No one can stop it. When the time comes, I'll try to organize the Army to help the peasant farmers with plowing and sowing."

My heart fills with joy. I look on him with admiration, exhilaration, and respect. He's a real Serb. He's a man who loves life. In the darkness of war, I'm fortunate enough to meet a man who is protecting our beleaguered hopes.

Once, when we were driving around Glina, I asked him to stop along the roadside so that I could pick a bouquet of daffodils. Flowers were growing in large clusters in the front yard of a deserted house. Marko stopped the car and I hopped out. I began picking flowers avidly until I noticed that the stems were standing at an angle because the ground had been disturbed. Someone had been digging here. I froze with terror at the thought that this terrain might have been mined. That killed the idea of picking any more flowers, so I slowly and cautiously retraced my exact steps back to the road.

The next day, a mine exploded in that same house. Several people were killed. I had almost been caught in the trap. I was shaken for days afterwards. Marko begged me not to torture myself with thoughts about what might have happened. Mines appeared everywhere as mushrooms do after a rainfall, and it's not easy to get rid of them. You simply have to be cautious, alert, and aware at all times for the telltale signs of enemy treachery — just as I was.

It's already the end of March 1993. Spring is coming. The war is still going on. One late afternoon, I was taking a cold-water bath when I heard the wail of ambulance sirens. I got dressed in a hurry and ran downstairs just as they were bringing in the patient. He had been shot in the head. Blood was streaming out. He was still conscious and he was saying, begging us: "Please don't shave my head!"

I shouted to the driver to prepare a car for Banja Luka. There wasn't a surgeon here who could perform a cranial operation to remove the bullet that had lodged in the right temple at the occipital bone. The entry wound was gushing blood and brain fragments. In the Surgical Outpatient Department, I intubated the patient, sedated him, and inserted a catheter. I helped Dr. Sara, who was with me all the time, bandage the wound. She had started her specialization in anesthesiology just as the war began, so she ended up spending only a year at the VMA. Then she was immediately thrust into the whirlwind of war. She lacked experience and knowledge, but she was already dealing with problems that would have challenged far more experienced anesthesiologists. I explained everything that I was doing, down to the smallest detail. She was quick on the uptake and she ended up being of great help.

While I was bandaging this unfortunate man's head, applying the required technique for this kind of injury, blood was soaking right through the bandages. My hands and scrubs were drenched in blood. The surgeon on duty called General Headquarters and requested a transport helicopter. I disagreed. Helicopter flights were prohibited without UNPROFOR permission, and that took twenty-four hours. This young man had no chance of surviving if we waited. It was already evening. Why risk the lives of two pilots and a helicopter for a dead man? If a helicopter took off without UNPROFOR permission, they could shoot it down. And even if they did get approval, there was still no guarantee that the helicopter wouldn't be fired on. This was one of the many situations in which it was so difficult for us to admit our powerlessness. We took in a living patient, and now we were going to watch him die because there was no chance of helping him. Such professional helplessness is horrifying. The patient was a young man who was born in 1963. He was tall, and he wore a chain around his neck with a cross, which bore the likeness of the Crucified Jesus Christ.

I called Velimir, the anesthetist, who was at home. He got here in five minutes and he didn't complain. He packed up everything he needed. I stabilized the patient's breathing and we took him to a waiting car. The door closed and they left. I stood there with my hands and scrubs drenched in blood. I was reeking of death. I washed in the bathtub, thinking all the while about the group that had just left. They could be hit by a grenade or meet up with a sniper or hit a mine anywhere along the way. I trembled at the thought, and still the patient had no chance of recovery. Yet it wasn't up to us to decide who lived or died. All too often, we were their last chance. We're risking the lives of our fellow doctors and nurses in order to give them that last fighting chance. But it's much more difficult to take responsibility for the lives of others. It would have been easier to divide myself into two people and to have gone to Banja Luka myself.

At the beginning of the war, the wounded were transported in large numbers by helicopter from Krajina to Belgrade. The nurses who volunteered to accompany them were thinking only of their patient's wellbeing, so they didn't take into consideration the inevitable problem of how to return to Krajina. The helicopter flights were only going in one direction, so the nurses often found themselves stranded in Serbia without any money and still wearing their bloodstained uniforms. There was no organized transportation. The great number of wounded patients had over-burdened the clinic's resources, so there was no one to look after the staff's basic needs. The nurses didn't want to bother anyone or beg, but there was no one to whom they could turn. So they started back to Glina on foot in their bloodstained uniforms. A seven-hundred kilometer journey lay ahead of them.

These nurses had left their children in Glina. Those children were all they had. They were happy to be alive. They met gracious, considerate people along the way who drove them across Serbia to the Bosnian border, and brought them to what was known as "the corridor" — a road Serbs had built so they could travel safely to Krajina, which was now in Croatia — and from there they went partly on foot or hitchhiked. They would arrive exhausted, filthy, hungry, and disoriented after about seven days. They would meet their supervisor in that condition, who would inquire tactlessly and arrogantly about where they had been. One exasperated nurse gave her supervisor a hard slap to the face. The unfortunate nurse was summarily fired. This was a completely inappropriate and needless display of authority. The hospital staff, headed by Dr. Dario, stood behind our distressed colleague until she was reinstated with financial compensation and a written apology.

* * * *

Vuković, a patient, calls us from the ICU:

"Doctor, Doctor! Help me!" he shouts. "I can't take the pain!!"

I reluctantly go to see him. What can I tell him? That I can't help him? He has to have another operation.

I sadly tell the nurses: "Put him to sleep. Give him pain-killers and put an oxygen mask on him. Let him at least sleep."

He falls asleep for a moment, but he wakes up again. The scene repeats itself. Dario was right when he told me not to get attached to patients. But what can I do? It's really difficult for him. Vuković is Croatian. He and his brother were with the Serbs from the very beginning when there were only twenty of them manning the barricades against their fellow Croats. The Croats had begun by limiting the Serbs' freedom of movement back in 1990. This inaugurated the next wave of persecution, which was the firing of Serbs *en masse* from their jobs. The Serbs protested by building barricades from tree trunks in the areas where they lived in order to prevent the Croatian police from arresting people simply for being Serbian. These two Croatian brothers had taken the side of the Serbs here in Glina.

Their mother had left them and gone over to the Croatian side. Vuković had just returned from the front and was cleaning his automatic rifle in the front yard of his home. He had forgotten a bullet was still in the chamber. The gun went off. The bullet went through his stomach, pancreas, spleen, and kidney. He was badly wounded. When they brought him in, he was in a state of shock, and it looked as if there wasn't a drop of blood left in him. Dario operated on him immediately without complications, but afterwards he warned us that the pancreas would cause problems on or about the seventh day after the operation. He was right. There was blood in both draining tubes, and there was blood on the probe, so he needed a second operation. The spleen was full of pus, which was flowing down into his stomach, and his abdomen was full of coagulating blood. I gave him a transfusion and fought the infection with massive doses of antibiotics.

Two days later, his condition remained unchanged. I pricked the central vein and I made a puncture in the pleura so that air could get in. I felt miserable. We tried to solve this problem by draining the rib cage. More pain was the last thing he needed.

Everyone loved him. Friends from his company came to see him. He received seven liters of blood from Serbs, so we joked that he was now a genuine Serb. Nationality didn't matter. Only the insane could justify pointless ethnocentrism. We worked hard to save patients regardless of their ethnicity. The Hippocratic Oath guides us.

My job is to save lives, not to kill. At the beginning of war, when the Army was still a united force, they brought wounded soldiers of different nationalities to Knin. Some were separatist enemies whose lives were in danger. After we resuscitated them, other soldiers would get angry.

"Why are you saving their lives? Why don't you just kill 'em?"

"Don't expect me to do your job," I retorted sharply to one soldier. "I'm a doctor, you idiot!"

We were indignant at the way these soldiers conducted themselves, so we asked the Colonel Dr. M. I. to keep them away from us. We're doctors. Anyone who comes to us with a chance of surviving is surely going to survive.

After these experiences, I began fearing retaliation, but nothing happened. Luckily, only a small percentage of the soldiers were as perverted as that one soldier who wanted me to kill a patient. Most of them understand the situation we're in. The Army collects blood for and from Muslim and Croat soldiers, as well.

Since we had to operate on patient Vuković again, I decided that he should be transported. Dr. Dario had by this time gone to Belgrade to get equipment and food, and I didn't have a single experienced surgeon here who could have solved this serious problem. I personally thought that there was another puncture in his stomach but I didn't have the right diagnostic tools to find out. I was sending him to Banja Luka according to the agreement with our colleagues there. As we were parting, I clasped his hand. He grabbed both my hands and wouldn't let go.

"Take care of yourself," I say.

"You too, Doctor. Take care. These days, the evils of war have the upper hand. It's no time for people," he shouts as they push his gurney towards the ambulance.

I feel tears welling up in my eyes. O, God am I losing my mind? I rush to the toilet. I take two deep breaths. It's over. Life goes on.

Patient Vuković was not operated on in Banja Luka. They felt that their staff was not sufficiently competent, so they transported him to Belgrade. I spent three days on the phone trying to find him. The hospital in Banja Luka transferred me to VMC (Military Medical Center), which then transferred me to the VMA. One of my colleagues there was persistent in searching the computer system, but she couldn't find him. Then I called the University Clinical Center. I called the First and then the Second Surgical Hospitals, but Vuković wasn't there, either. His brother comes to see me every day. He has to walk fifteen kilometers in each direction.

"I don't know what to do, Doctor. My aunt died yesterday. Our mother has left us. My father died. Is my brother going to make it?"

His quiet voice left no room for consolation. He gave me his hand when we were saying good-bye. I held it tightly as if I could somehow relieve his sadness and pain. He's a Croat fighting on the side of the Serbs. Croatia has just declared its independence and has violently seceded from Yugoslavia. Serbs want to preserve the country in its entirety, and this is especially true for the Serbs that live in multi-national communities. Croatian nationalist authorities abhor Serbs, so they deprive them of their right to be a constitutionally equal party in the citizenry of their new country, despite the fact that Serbs have lived in these territories for at least five hundred years.

Croats who live with Serbs have, in most cases, shown solidarity with their neighbors, as is the case with the Vuković brothers. In Serbia, the notion of nationality is irrelevant. The wounded all receive the same treatment regardless of nationality.

I was tireless in my pursuit. I had to find Vuković even if he were dead. My duty is to honor his solidarity. On Friday morning, I finally reached the head of the medical corps at the VMC in Banja Luka. I had given up hope.

"Good morning, Colonel Karjanović."

"Good morning Doctor, how are you?" he says, somewhat warmly.

This gives me a spark of hope.

"I wonder if you could help me. I have been looking for a patient for days," I stammer, surprised by his kindness.

"I was advised of your persistence," he continues in the same tone of voice. "He's the first on the list for KBC (Clinical Hospital Center "Dragiša Mišović" in the Belgrade), in the Surgical Intensive Care Department."

"Thank you!" I say almost apologetically.

"Where are you from, Doctor?" he asks.

"From Serbia, from Belgrade! I'm a volunteer from Serbia," I say as the words come tumbling out. "I'm looking out for a patient, a Croat. I must do my duty and follow up his recovery."

"I applaud you, Doctor. Every patient's life is important. I appreciate that. Whenever you come to Banja Luka, stop by for a cup of coffee."

"Colonel, I'll come by as soon as this war ends," I say with a laugh.

"Exactly! Bless you," he replies.

We said good-bye. Perhaps one day I'm going to join him for that cup of coffee in Banja Luka, after all.

PART TWO

16. The Whirlwind of Destiny

When I wake up in the morning on the second floor of the hospital in Glina, I can see through the window the tops of pine trees: here whitened by snow, there green, and all bedashed by quietly drizzling rain. A few people are scurrying about with umbrellas.

Spring is coming.

Here in Krajina, we come across so many different types of uniforms that I'm unable to distinguish their insignia. One patient's uniform resembles an American one, but the state flag is not easy to discern. Uniforms for the Territorial Defense Forces of Krajina are also diverse and they represent a combination of different Yugoslav Army uniforms. Volunteers arriving in Krajina have been trained by the JNA, so they are prepared to deal with any situation they might encounter. There is also a smaller number of organized groups, which together with the JNA and the Territorial Defense, represents a substantial and well organized military force. Last, but not least, there are small-time criminals and ideologues from Serbia who've had no prior military training or combat experience, and who have brought their own weapons. Unfortunately, these volunteers outnumber all the others.

Most of the wounded soldiers who are brought in are unarmed, so I seldom see weapons. Once a wounded soldier is admitted, he becomes my patient. I'm not interested in what uniform or symbols a he may be wearing, nor am I interested to which group he may belong. The wounded soldiers I encounter have already had their uniforms removed during the administration of first aid, which is also true for those soldiers who are our enemies at this moment in history. The only general conclusion I can draw about the uniforms my patients wear is that they fit badly.

One afternoon a surgeon, along with another volunteer, called me into his office to meet someone whom he described as "an interesting person." Everyone knows that I'm keeping a diary, so they try to introduce me to as many "interesting people" as possible. When I came into the room, I was almost breathless with surprise. Standing in front of me was a tall, exceptionally handsome young man, perhaps my own age. He wore a uniform that had many pockets. He had left his weapons leaning against the wall. He was outfitted like a sniper.

Grrr... I thought as my entire body reacted viscerally to his presence. *Stay away from me!* This guy is scaring the hell out of me.

The Sniper, as he was known, was supposed to be a member of a special military unit, but I didn't know which one, so I didn't know on whose side he was fighting. His eyes were blue-grey. He moved with great poise yet he appeared cold. We shook hands, exchanged hardly a word or two, and then the conversation ended. I felt something unpleasant in my bones, so I quickly said good-bye and left. Later, I saw him talking to the Director. They were examining a sheaf of documents.

The next day, in the early evening when I was relaxing in my room after an exhausting day, someone knocked on my door. Without even waiting for me to answer, Dr. Aleksandar, the surgeon, barged into my room with the Sniper. He explained that two raiding parties had been apprehended. The atmosphere suddenly became tense. No one could predict when an attack might occur. The Sniper wanted to take us to a shooting range for target practice. I, however, did not want to use a firearm. No matter how skillful I may be, I wasn't going to stand much of a chance in a showdown with a professional.

Dr. Aleksandar disagreed. He had gotten a gun for self-defense, even though weapons cannot be purchased legally without a special permit in Glina. Everything is under military control. I like that. I feel safer here than I did in Knin. They're actually looking out for us here. But now I felt that I could no longer protest, because I would have been attracting unwanted attention. So I agreed to go to the shooting range. On the way there, however, the Sniper and his friends unexpectedly changed their plans. We ended up making a detour to some pub. (Pubs were not allowed to operate, so this one had its windows covered.) The men I was with didn't say a word. No one questioned the change of plan. I also said nothing. It was already dark. We stayed at the pub for about an hour. I was tired, and would have gladly gone back to my room to sleep, but my companions weren't even going to consider going back yet.

We played pool and managed to relax a little. I don't know anything about the game, but I had some beginner's luck. By coincidence, or perhaps by design, my partner in this game was the Sniper. People were keeping their distance from him. He dealt with my mistakes, and then we started winning. Tall and limber, he stalked the pool table like a predator. He could lean over it and sink a ball into a far pocket. He showed off his mastery of the game by mixing straight and bank shots. He tried to meet my eyes before and after every shot, which made it seem as though he wanted approval or recognition. I was never particularly skilled at being coy with men, so I avoided his gaze. He'd squeeze my hand from time to time. I remained silent and pretended that I hadn't noticed. My colleagues from the hospital seemed to enjoy seeing this strange guy come on to me. I got the impression that I was being set up. Even if the Sniper were flirting, I wouldn't have known how to react without hurting his feelings. He gave me the creeps.

There was also another man in our group whom I hadn't seen before. He was tall and unshaven and he had long hair. He was wearing a green camouflage uniform that bore no clear markings. He mingled with the doctors and nurses, and played a few games with them. They never introduced him to me.

After the game, when we were sitting at a corner table, the Sniper took my hand again. "I came here tonight because of you!" he said. "There's something I want to tell you. I want you to listen to me," he added, speaking quickly and indistinctly.

I wasn't being paranoid, after all, I thought. The Sniper didn't end up shooting a game of pool with me by accident. Since he already seemed friendly with my colleagues, I figured that he was a friend. His eyes were shining feverishly. I saw a troubled soul, so the doctor in me reacted immediately and I began feeling sorry for him. Who knows what's bothering him? I thought. There are plenty of others like him.

"All right, that's why I'm here," I said. "I'm listening. Go on"

"I can't talk here," the Sniper replied in a low voice. "Let's talk someplace else."

We finally left in a dilapidated two-door Zastava 101 to go back to the hospital. The stranger in the camouflage uniform joined us. He wasn't untidy, but he had an unkempt beard and his hair was longer than what we normally saw. His eyes were bloodshot and he looked a little confused. It was pitch-dark already. The curfew was in effect. Policemen stopped us, looked into the car, and then recognized my companion. Then they waved us through. I was wondering why he didn't need an official pass. It was strange to see him enjoying such privileges. We arrived at the hospital. I was sitting in the front passenger seat next to the Sniper, while his friend was sitting in the back seat behind me. I'd have to get out of the car to let him out. I waited for the Sniper to get out, too. But he remained in the driver's seat, and he urged me to get back into the car so we could talk.

His friend stepped away from the car. Then he suddenly seized my hand. He drew me close to him.

"Doctor, I have to tell you something," he said. "Let me explain. I can't feel anything toward people. I simply can't. How can a dead man feel emotions? Maybe I'm crazy, but I can still tell that you're an exceptional woman. You had enough guts to come to this fucking hell hole to help us any way you can — but no one can help us."

He turned grim and menacing again.

"We're killers!" he continued. "How can a man go on living who was taught not to kill — but has killed?"

He snarled and howled in anguish.

He was frightening me. I slowly walked backward toward the car, where the Sniper was waiting for me.

"I killed a man and then I died myself," he said, continuing his confession. "I slaughtered a man in cold blood.... Look ... look at my hands! They're still bloody!"

He shoved his hands under my nose.

"Smell the blood!" he said in a rasping voice as his eyes grew glassy and distant. "I killed a Croat, but he was a human being, too. Hey, I'm not insane. Everyone is going to tell you that I'm insane. But I just have that damn feeling because of my guilty conscience. I'm thinking: *That's the problem!* One shouldn't think too much in a war. You can't turn into an animal if you aren't one already, right? But I killed, and then I died that very same moment. There's no drug, no brandy, no sleep that will help me forget the blood — the dead."

I held his hand and tried to speak but the words were caught in my throat. I was afraid I was going to say something wrong. What could I have said to him anyway?!

"What are you going to say to me?" he asked, seeing the difficulty I was having to speak. "Nothing. I'm too far gone. When I disappear from the face of this earth, everyone'll be relieved. Seeing how others react when they start killing is the only thing that keeps me going. Everyone's gotta know that murder doesn't go unpunished.

"I'm crazy, see? So what! Let 'em all see that I'm kill-crazy. They better watch out, Doc. I'm a dead man walking. Nothing you or anybody else can do about it. It's too late for me. I can't fall in love with you or anyone else. And I would love to be able to love again.

"I hate myself," he continued, sighing. "But I admire you, lady. Thank you for arousing feelings in me that are bringing me back to this shitty world. You doctors are the only ones who don't treat us like murderers. You like us motherfuckers. That's all we need: someone to love us in this fucking strange world. O, dying like this hurts so much...."

Finally he started walking unsteadily towards the hospital. He was armed to the teeth. I was on the verge of tears when I came back into the car again. I was shaking. The car engine was idling and making a quiet buzzing sound. The tears now running down my face prevented me from seeing the Sniper's face — all I could see were his hands on the steering wheel.

"Aren't you afraid to be with him?" I asked the Sniper.

"Why should I be afraid of him? He's harmless," I said.

"He's good for nothing now," said the Sniper. "He used to be one of Krajina's preeminent intellectuals. When the war started, he stayed here because he honestly wanted to help, while plenty of others in his position fled. There was no military force here to protect the locals. The local Territorial Defense kept transferring him from one place to another. He didn't complain. His country — his home, which meant everything to him, was being attacked by Croats. Everything he loved had been endangered. It was logical that he, as a man, would want to protect it.

"Once, we were passing through a village that had been ravaged by a squad of Croatian convicts. We found a whole family slaughtered, from the baby all the way to grandma and grandpa. The sight of it sickened us. We were screaming, writhing in pain on the ground. That was when we snapped. We were roaring like wild beasts. Why did they have to kill these people?! It would have been easier for me if they had cut out my eyes. I'm a fighter. I'm up to facing challenges in war. But this killing of civilians — children — completely dehumanized us. The mounting rage ... fury ... misery ... despair.... All I wanted to do was kill ... kill! And kill we did! We slaughtered innocents, too, in the first Croatian village we found. They were just as innocent as our victims were.

"Fuck war. You gotta show 'em that they can't go killing just like that and walk away scot-free. We have to fight fire with fire. If you're honest, you go ahead and make the sacrifice. Then you go insane. Wars aren't for anybody who's got any brains at all. War's for idiots. I admire you. You know what war is, but you still came here to help us."

I was staring through the windshield. Everything was dark. I was hypnotized by the sound of the Sniper's his voice. From the corner of my eye, I saw his hands moving up and down as he stroked the steering wheel, talking all the while. His voice changed in depth and intensity. An icy fear was congealing inside me, choking me. I felt like I was freezing. I had to get out of there.

I stepped with one foot out of the car and held the door with one hand while shifting my weight from the seat to my leg outside the car.

"Don't go!" he cried. "I want to tell you something. I have to talk to someone. I have to ask you something."

He seized my arm and yanked me with tremendous force back into the car.

"All right ... all right.... Tell me what it is," I said, returning to the seat.

My patience was strained to the limit, but it was clear that he needed me. He took my hand gently and drew me close to him. I rebuffed him but not rudely.

"I can't breathe." I said, in as level a voice as I could summon. "Let me see your eyes. What is it? I am listening."

He turned abruptly and started the car. It lurched forward. The guards let him pass again and we plunged into the darkness.

I could hear distant machine-gun fire. I didn't know where we were we going. I started trembling again but remained silent. I was starting to realize that I was in a car with a mentally disturbed man and that there was no one around to help me. The guards had given him a free pass. He was privileged; I was alone. I thought about jumping out of the car but the door couldn't be opened from the inside on the passenger side, so there was no way out. I was dreading all the possible things that might happen to me. He was roaring down the streets like a lunatic, and he kept talking to himself. I couldn't make sense of what he was saying because of the engine noise, but even if I could have heard what he was saying, I probably wouldn't have been able to understand what he was talking about anyway.

Terrified, I began entertaining grim fantasies. My poor children! They would be left motherless. I was going to die in the most miserable possible way. I only hoped that it would be quick — without torture. He was armed: he had a knife with a serrated edge in his boot and a gun in his holster. Was he going to torture me?

Suddenly he braked the car, stopping sharply.

"You're not asking me anything?" he shouted angrily.

I was silent. I trembled.

"Take me back to the hospital. Something might happen. There might be an emergency case. I'm the only anesthesiologist," I said, grasping at straws.

He said nothing. As suddenly as he had stopped, he started driving again. Soon he stopped again on a side street near the deserted ruins of buildings. It was completely dark. Nothing was visible. There was no one around. We were alone. Maybe he was going to rape me. I didn't care about being raped. I was afraid he was going to kill me. Fear was getting the better of me. I couldn't speak. I suspected that I wouldn't survive. I tasted blood in my mouth. I had bitten my cheek.

"Tell me, who's that Vrcelj guy?" he growled. "Who's he working for?"

"What do you mean? He's an officer. The Army pays him," I said through clenched teeth and bloody sputum.

"Don't hand me that shit. Why did he commandeer that truck? Who's paying him? Let's have it! You don't pull stunts like that and then go scot-free."

I said nothing because I knew nothing. What could I have said, since Marko never mentioned anything about a truck, let alone any details about his operations. I finally understood that I was being kidnapped for information about Colonel Vrcelj!

I was in a state of shock. The Sniper slapped me around. Then he pounced on me with the force of a tiger. He pushed me across the fixed seat. My back bent unnaturally. The weight of his forearm was pressing against my throat. He was chocking me! I was trying to resist, to get away but there was no place to go. The more I struggled against him, the harder he leaned on my throat until I could no longer breathe. He was muscular, and he stood over six feet tall. I felt my bones cracking. If only the seat were lower! I was afraid he was going to break my back. My head was thrown so far back that I was suffocating. I was struggling for air, slowly losing consciousness. I would have gladly escaped my body in order to avoid what followed.

I was no longer in my body. He could torture my body but he couldn't touch my mind. I sank into a mist where I could see red spheres and I heard the dirges of a funeral liturgy. My soul was leaving my body. I saw it as a thin red-yellow line rising upward. I had the impression someone had hung me on a hook and was hoisting me upward. I was unable to resist.

With my last bit of energy, I looked at my legs, which had been squeezed and pressed by his. I saw the gear shift rammed into my thigh, which was hurting me. I knew that it was going to leave a big bruise if I managed to survive. My mind was detached and I was wondering: what's the purpose of all this? What had Marko done? I didn't even know Marko that well. Why did he need me if he was after Marko? Why was this horrible man holding me to blame?

I lost consciousness. Red circles alternated with black ones in hot waves. Between the red circles, I saw a black knife blade tearing open my stomach and ripping upwards to my throat. Everything hurt. The pain protected me from dying. I knew that I was still alive as long as I felt pain.

I regained consciousness with my face buried in a heap of dirty snow behind the hospital. That was where he had dumped me. It was cold. I was afraid I was frostbitten. My fingers were stiff and twisted. I couldn't move them. Still in shock, I irrelevantly wondered what I looked like. I shifted my position. The pain coursing through my entire body reminded me of what had happened earlier. I didn't dare think about it. If I had, I would have screamed. And if I had screamed, I would have attracted attention, and then I would have to explain what happened. I didn't want to see anyone. I didn't want to explain anything to anyone. All of a sudden, I wanted to die. I wanted to disappear. I felt my body and I was relieved to find that I still had my clothes on. I was still alive. I wasn't going to think about anything. I wasn't going to think.

I got up slowly. It was still night. The hospital was shrouded in darkness. Here and there you could see the glimmering light of a candle. No one could see me. I came up to the entrance as slowly and as quietly as I could, and I painfully climbed the stairs to my floor, praying that I wouldn't run into anyone. I crept into my room and found a towel. I needed to take a bath but there was no hot water, so I sat in a tub of ice-cold water. Everything between my legs was swollen and bloody. It was painful. The chaos in my mind hurt even more. All of a sudden, outrage began welling within me, and it slowly overcame me. The coloration of my body was changing from black to blue to reddishness as if it were in the grip of tentacles. I wanted to scream. I wanted to lash out at everything around me. Then I remembered that it was night, and that I mustn't awaken anyone. No one should see me in this condition. I clutched the wash basin tightly as if I wanted to discharge all my aggression into it. I was snarling, shaking my head as if I were shouting: No... No... No!

As I was gnashing my teeth, I felt a sharp pain in my jaw. I felt pain in my ears. Blood filled my mouth again. I raised my head. My throat was tense with unspoken words. My eyes were wide open. Tears came streaming down my cheeks. I felt the warmth of my tears. I was on my knees, still furiously clutching the wash basin. I imagined pitching it across the room. I imagined myself crashing it against the wall and destroying everything in my absolute fury. I felt an outburst of anger so violent that I fell on the bathroom floor and — was it for several minutes? — trembled there like a wounded animal.

Writhing in pain, I refused to accept reality. I suddenly became afraid that I would pass out on the bathroom floor and that someone would find me here naked. I got up with my last atom of strength. Then I somehow felt lighter. I sat down again in the cold water and waited for the injured parts of my body to go numb so that I could touch the wounds and wash them. I got dressed and went to my room. I occasionally felt some surges of heat through my frozen body. Waves of heat came from somewhere, warming me and easing my pain. That helped me pull myself together. These sensations were protecting me from the outer world. Everything still hurt, but somehow less so. I felt open wounds throbbing throughout my entire body, and I felt the irrational fear that they were going to start bleeding and that everyone was going to be able to see them. Suddenly, I felt ashamed. I couldn't tell anyone about this. I felt so ashamed. Ashamed! Why didn't I run away when we were still near the hospital? Why did I trust him? I wanted to scream again but I knew that I mustn't. Tears kept rolling down my face.

When I entered my room, Dara woke up and said sleepily: "Sarah, you know you can't run with the hares and hunt with the hounds. What will Marko say? What were you doing with that spy?"

"It's okay, Dara." I say weakly, "I'm not cheating on Marko. How do you know that the Sniper is a spy?"

"He's a Croat, you know. God himself only knows who he's working for. You'd better stay away from him. There's something fishy about this whole business. Up there where the borders of Croatia, Bosnia and Krajina meet, trucks with contraband cigarettes and gasoline are going across our territory into Croatia. There's been something going on over there for the past few days. Everyone is upset and the situation is tense. I heard that Marko confiscated several trucks. The people are happy because he's doing that. You better watch out!"

"Don't worry, Dara. He and his friend just needed someone to talk to. That's all," I said. "They need a psychiatrist. I guess I function here as a psychologist-psychiatrist, as well, so I listen to what people have to say. Everyone's having a hard time, Dara. You know that. Everyone's a little crazy. I finally realized that. I'm really tired. I'm going to sleep now. Please don't wake me in the morning unless it's an emergency."

Exhausted and worried, I try to figure out what was going on. Are they going to kill Marko? Is what happened tonight supposed to be a warning to him? I don't mean anything to them. I'm just a doctor, a volunteer. Marko is an enigma to the enemy. If he has indeed confiscated their merchandise, as Dara said, then he is putting them out of business. They have to stop him, but they first have to find out who was standing behind him before they can kill him. Was I beaten and humiliated simply to send him a message? His son could be next! I stiffen with worry and shame. Despite being plagued these thoughts, I managed to fall asleep.

I awake at noon. Dara didn't awaken me. It seems as though there's no work to do. I get up cautiously and inspect my body. My face is puffy but it has no visible bruises. My legs are streaked by black and blue marks. Going to the toilet is torture. I groan. I take antibiotics as well as analgesics. I'm so weak that bacteria could easily attack my compromised immune system. No one must notice that I am in pain. After I get dressed, I think, no one will notice anything.

Marko calls. He says that he's going to Knin for two weeks. He doesn't have time to visit me to say good-bye. He's going to call later from Knin. That's all right. There's no reason to tell him about what happened. I have to go through this alone. If the Sniper's goal is to alarm Marko and provoke a response, then that's not going to happen. Marko isn't going to know anything about this. By the time he returns, the bruises shall have vanished, and he'll be none the wiser. There's no reason for anyone to know anything about this. I have to keep the whole situation under control. I'm not going to let the Sniper win. My tears mingle with pain and anger. I'm half dead but I still have to put on a happy face. It's not that difficult, actually, because so many others here are doing the same: the happy-faced walking dead.

The days passed and I didn't see the Sniper. I didn't dare make any inquiries, but I did try to find out whether anyone had said anything about him. Instead of talking about *him*, everyone was discussing Marko, who had confiscated a truckload of black-market cigarettes that was on its way to Croatia. And then he impounded a fuel tanker truck. The people were grateful to him. I was proud of Marko, but I was also afraid for his life. All this makes me feel that something terrible is going to happen.

Marko returned after two weeks, but we saw each other only briefly. He was complaining about organized crime, which had become a serious problem in Krajina. The worst thing about it was the compelling reasons that led one to believe that members of the Army were involved in it. Marko couldn't tell which way the wind was blowing. He had some suspicions about who might be involved in black-market gasoline, cigarettes, and vehicles, but he had no way of putting a stop to it. The local gangs were against him, so he had to fight them with everything he had. I kept my mouth shut. I didn't say a word about my encounter with the Sniper. I only begged Marko to be careful.

* * * *

A few days later they sent me to the neighboring town of Vojnić where we had to perform an operation. There were no anesthesiologists there. The nurse anesthetist who had worked in Vojnić returned to Serbia. I went on the trip with surgeons who had arrived only a month earlier. We performed the operation, and then we all went to have a meal in the dining room. The Director wanted to show me how they had managed to convert a motel into an improvised hospital. We turned the Health Center in Glina into a wartime hospital, but that wasn't as difficult as turning a motel into a hospital. Motel rooms are unsuitable as either operating rooms or sterilization facilities, so we felt a great deal of respect for those who managed to carry on in wartime conditions. I had mentioned earlier that the first hospital on Serbian territory in Croatia was in Petrova Gora. A year after the war had begun, the hospital personnel were divided into two groups: one left for Glina (Banija); while the other remained here in Vojnić (Kordun), where they repurposed a motel. These two groups cooperated occasionally, as they're doing now.

Buoyed by a feeling of admiration, I set off with Dr. D—, the Hospital Director. He was an otolaryngologist, a doctor who specializes in diseases connected with the ear and throat. He was in charge of the improvised hospital, which had two other doctors on the staff. There was an OR and a Pharmacy. That was all I knew about it. First, Dr. D— took me to his office. I cast curious glances as I entered with him. On the table, there were tangerines, Coca-Cola, and chocolates. These items came from the duty-free zone. It had been a long time since I'd seen — let alone enjoyed — such delicacies. The Serbian Orthodox Church was sending them humanitarian aid, but it was systematically overlooking to send aid to our group in Glina. After we entered his office, he suddenly locked the door behind him, which I didn't like: an alarm bell went off in my head. He turned, looked at me angrily, seized me by my shoulders, and began shaking me violently: "What are you doing down there in Banija? What's your pal Vrcelj doing? Who's backing him up?"

I was paralyzed with shock. What was the matter with him?

While I was trying to push him away, the door opened with a bang and the Sniper burst into the room. He had a MIG 22 rifle in his hands. The sight of him alarmed me. Run! I thought. The instinct was stronger than the pounding of my heart. I ducked cat-like past the gun-wielding Sniper, and ran down the corridor. I didn't look back. I felt my heart was going to leap into my throat. I knew he wasn't going to shoot. He already could have killed me if he had wanted to. I ran into the dining room where my colleagues were at table. Steaming-hot fried potatoes, which we didn't have in Glina, were being served. There were onions, cheese and, of course, Coca Cola. I wasn't hungry, but I quickly joined the group and I started eating. They were laughing and talking, so no one was paying any attention to me. No one noticed that I was out of breath and upset.

Immediately after I sat down, Dr. D— entered the dining room. He was red in the face. He didn't even bother to look at me. The Sniper was nowhere to be seen. I stared silently at my plate. I finished eating and then went quickly to the car that was going back to Glina. It was already dark. Few stars were visible in the night sky. The moon was breaking through heavy, black clouds. I was shivering even though my companions were saying that it wasn't really that cold. I threw my coat over my shoulders. I tried to fall asleep. All of a sudden at a bend in the road, our minibus began to slow down. In front of us stood the Sniper, who had emerged from the shadows and was waving us to a stop. Everyone seemed to know him and a friendly murmur arose. Our vehicle came to a stop and the door opened. He loomed in the doorway talking loudly over the engine noise:

"Hey guys, I hope that you won't mind if I *borrow* the Doc for a while. I need her to solve a problem for us. I'll bring her right back. Some anesthesia equipment has arrived, so we need some help with it."

They opened the door so I could get out. I remained silent, wondering whether my colleagues had set me up. This was the second time that they were delivering me into his hands. The first time had been at the pub. Did they know what had happened to me? They must have. I was certain there was a conspiracy. I became paranoid. At that moment, I hated each and every one of them. These were people I worked with every day and it turned out that I couldn't trust them. Even so, the possibility existed that they may not have known anything at all. I kept my mouth shut. I just sat down in the car with the Sniper. What did he want now? Was he going to assault me again? I turned rigid with resistance. I wasn't going to show him that I was afraid. I wasn't going to let him humiliate me again.

I presumed that the Sniper was not going to kill me because he needed me alive in order to blackmail Marko. I didn't think he would rape me again, either. He wouldn't be able to throw me into the snow behind the hospital now, since everyone saw that it was he who asked me to join him. My colleagues would be thinking that he really needed me for the equipment that had allegedly just arrived. Maybe they thought we were interested in each other. Maybe some of them were against Marko and would somehow benefit if he were out of the way. It was all about Marko. I didn't matter. I had to figure this out. I was afraid, but protecting Marko was more important, so I had to endure what was about to happen.

My colleagues drove nonchalantly away, and left me alone with my tormentor. He drove to a ledge by the road and there he parked the car in the dark. Bright moon broke through the clouds and flooded us with light. The few stars twinkling above appeared to be mocking me with their optimism.

I didn't even look at my tormentor. I didn't want to. I couldn't. I was ashamed. I was a victim but I almost felt guilty because he had assaulted me. I sat and waited, petrified. He got out of the car and started hitting the roof angrily. I remained silent, thinking again of my children. Tears welled up in my eyes uncontrollably. This frightening loneliness and constant danger were killing me slowly.

He got into the car again. I heard him crying. It was a kind of low moan. He leaned towards me. I tried to move away from him banging on the car door. He reached out, took my trembling shoulders, and pulled me close to him. My nose pressed against the sharp edges of the pockets of his military uniform. He held me tightly like a child and started to cry again. He sobbed bitterly.

"I know that I'm asking too much," he said. "But I beg you to forgive me if you can."

He gazed at me pleadingly.

"I've gone crazy. I've got no excuse. All of us are kind of crazy. I beg you to forgive me for what I did. I made a big, big mistake in my judgment of you and Colonel Vrcelj. I'm not your enemy, although I must appear to be. I wanted to warn him. I got orders to investigate what he was doing and to send him a message to stop doing what he was doing. They told me that he was a crook and high jacking their goods. After I made inquiries, I found out that he was the only one who was being honest all along. I made a mistake … I was wrong. Please forgive me."

He relaxed a little, and then he reclined in his seat.

"I was angry with you. I liked you the first time I saw you. Then I heard that you were with him and that you might be taking part in his activities. I wanted to punish him — and you, too. But I was wrong. I hurt the only person who deserved any respect in all this chaos. I hurt you. You're innocent. I really feel terrible. This meeting tonight was a set-up. Dr. D— set a trap for you. Your colleagues in Glina have nothing to do with it. They're good guys and I told them I liked you. Don't hold them responsible for what's happened. Locals have their own rules around here. I knew that and the least I could do was to save you from that deranged idiot."

He stared through the windshield into the distance.

"Now, they'll try again to get to Colonel Vrcelj through you and his son to punish him, to try to stop him. You and his son are his vulnerabilities. They'll try to get to him. Everyone quickly found out about your relationship with him, so people started talking about you. They said that you'd softened up his attitude. All three of you have to leave Krajina as soon as possible. I'll let you know if I find out anything that might help you. You must find it hard to believe me, but this is the only thing I can do to redeem myself. I've caused you enough pain.

"While I was shadowing you because of Colonel Vrcelj's activities, I experienced a deep emotional catharsis. I was in turmoil."

He gripped the steering wheel again.

"Who's that woman who caught his fancy?" he said as his knuckles went white. "He's my enemy and so is this woman. In time, as I got to know you and kept hearing about you from your colleagues, I realized that the situation was not so simple. I realized that you were an idealist.

"The first word that comes to mind to describe your behavior is FOOLISH! You're a real fool, you know that? What are you doing here where you could get yourself killed over a single word? You say thousands of words every single day and any one of them can put you in danger! And you're doing it without even realizing what could happen. How can you be so blind to the darkness around you?"

"I've seen a lot here," I muttered. "My patients may or may not be responsible for corruption. I'm not asking you for anything. You don't have to be grateful to me. I just want my life, nothing else. I'm a doctor. I just came here to do my job. I'm not interested in anything else, and I don't want to understand anything else. I don't care about your local conflicts. I figured out that you were shadowing the ringleader of the local criminal gang. And you were shadowing Marko, too."

I felt my courage returning.

"I don't give a damn about that," I said. "Every confrontation has its tough guys, and there are even more confrontations during wartime. People don't live under the same conditions. As they say, it's war for some, profit for others. That's never going to change. So, I'm not interested in who pays you or who sent you. I simply don't want to know. The less I know, the better off I am. My only concern is to heal these poor people."

"We're repulsive," he groaned.

I protested. I didn't understand why I kept talking to this person who was getting weirder by the minute. My desire to protect Marko was greater than my fear. I didn't understand the boundaries. I would have endured anything to protect the man I loved. He enjoyed my respect, especially for the way he dealt with bullies. It was so hard to be decent in this filthy war. Marko had proved his decency beyond the shadow of doubt.

"We're no more repulsive than other people," protested the Sniper. "For God's sake, man! Neither of us have anybody we can trust. Where else in the world can you speak in your own language? Where? Is there any place on earth where you could actually be happy? I don't think so."

He was desperate, and he was practically screaming now. He was frightening me again. I felt myself blocking sensory experience as if I were giving up my ghost.

But he didn't assault me. He just kept on talking:

"Damn them all. People are starving and these animals are trafficking humanitarian aid. You have no idea. I'm working with them but they make me sick. I would kill them all but they're also my people. Who are we, anyway? We're all pathetic. I wonder if there's any chance of getting off this road to hell we've taken. It's disappearing behind us. Then I meet one person in this abominable shithole who reminds me that everything is not hopeless. You're a desert mirage! That's what you are. A mirage!"

What was he talking about? I thought. He's out of his mind! This man hurt me both physically and emotionally to punish Marko. He used the fact that I loved Marko to manipulate me. He could have threatened me; he could have beaten me; but why did he rape me? What was going on inside of his traumatized head? He was confusing his role in the war with his pre-war identity. We were all different people before the war. Trauma erases the difference between the professional and the private side of our personalities. A person becomes confused and vulnerable.

Deep inside, I knew I no longer understood the boundaries of socially acceptable conduct; otherwise, I would not have been sitting here with this thug.

"Who told you I'm so selfless?" I protested. "I'm here to save lives."

"My life is miserable," he continued quietly. "It didn't used to be so miserable — but now...."

"Get out of here. You'll live better and you'll be free," I advised him.

"Where can I go? I was born here. How would I then be able to return after the war and live normally? How can I leave others to fight in my place?"

"Nonsense," I scoffed. "You know as well as I do that there are plenty who ran away who've still got the brassbound nerve to return and make money again just as if nothing had ever happened. That's life."

"They'll be put on trial," he said.

"Who is going to bring anyone to trial? The government's up for sale right now, as it is during all wars."

He looked at me, almost laughing.

"Do you know how much I love you at this moment?" he asked. "You know what's going on, but you're still here."

He was confusing his roles again. The soldier in him was receding, so his pre-war personality was becoming dominant.

"I've got nowhere else to go. Krajina is my destiny," I whispered.

I felt hot tears welling up in my eyes.

"Tough," he said pathetically.

"I don't know if it's tough or not. It's what it is. It's hard for everyone."

"Look at the sky!" he exclaimed in a boyish and unexpectedly cheerful outburst.

The clouds were breaking up, but then they gathered again, and between them stars were twinkling. One star shined brighter than the others. "That's you, a star!" he said. "I'd like to run off with you, take you somewhere far away and keep you only for myself."

He paused, then disgorged another torrent of words.

"You didn't say anything to Vrcelj to save him. I could tell from the way he acted when we met. If he had known, he would have tried to kill me. You knew that, so you kept it to yourself. Everyone needs a confessor. If you're absolved of your wrong-doings — then you're forgiven."

"Please, let's go back to the hospital," I said. "Something could have happened but no one knows where I am."

I was still afraid of him. My body hadn't forgotten the suffering that he inflicted on it.

"None of them could care less about you or me!" he said bitterly.

"My coming here was a revolt, my plea to put an end this atrocity. Yes, it's dangerous and unprofitable. No one cares. But I'm an anesthesiologist, not a psychologist. You need someone more qualified than I am," I said as gently as I could.

He wept again. His face was on my neck. His tears were streaming down my breasts. I was exhausted and miserable. I was holding the head of a killer, a torturer, a low life, a has-been. I felt sorry for him. The doctor, as well as the human being in me, had forgiven him. What was going to happen next? He was mumbling in English and in Serbian. He had spent time abroad, so English came naturally to him.

"You have to believe me. I didn't kill children. I'm not capable of doing something like that. I just couldn't. If I had, then a bullet in the forehead would be the only way out for me. It'd be salvation from these nightmares."

"Are you going to commit suicide?" I asked.

"Who knows? I'll fight my own war. Hold me tight, so that I can feel you are here," he said and moaned so grievously that his pain penetrated me.

It was an existential pain that crept under your skin and lodged itself in your bones. We would never be free of it. I clasped my arms tightly around the man who almost killed me.

We sat in the car silently, as if we had been mummified. Our tears blurred the moon and stars that were still visible through the windshield.

He finally drove me back to the hospital. As soon as I got out of the car, I ran to my room. I was grateful that Dara, my room-mate, also a doctor, was not there. I wouldn't have had the ener-gy for any small talk, especially not for lying. I went to bed fully dressed and without having eaten. I fell into a morbid sleep. It seemed as if the dome of the sky had collapsed, and that we were surrounded by darkness. Now I knew how these people felt. There was no escape. The falling rubble from the dark dome of the sky had buried them, too.

I didn't recover from the shock of this encounter until days afterward. Questions arise and crowd my mind faster than I can answer them. How many of these poor devils are going to harm innocent people? Is there salvation? I just keep working and keep my mouth shut.

I really need to learn about psychotherapy. I don't want to make a mistake in dealing with people who have been deranged by suffering. I called my professor from postgraduate studies in psycho-physiology to seek his advice. He wasn't available, but his wife helped me. She's a psychiatrist who's working with people in Belgrade who returned from the front lines.

"I know exactly how you feel," she said. "You chose to be there, so you can't completely protect yourself. But don't worry. In most cases, these people were normal before the war. Their situational neurosis can often be cured by confidence and love. Rest assured that they feel and know instinctively who loves and understands them. That, in itself, is sometimes all they need. Sometimes it's more important than having a qualified psychia-trist. Love them, and you won't make a mistake. Give them a feeling of security and stability, a sense of being protected. That's what they desperately need."

It's true. They're looking for security. I'm looking for it, too. If I didn't love these people, then I wouldn't have left everything behind to come here. I understand them. I don't know when all this is going to end, and I am saddened by the fact that I can't love them all, listen to them all, and help them all. I'm insignificant but my sorrow is limitless.

After this last encounter, I only met the Sniper a handful of times. He kept his word, and he informed me about anything that might have put me or those close to me in danger. On one occasion, I was preparing to travel to Perna with the Director, Dr. Dario. We were going to visit his mother. It's an old Serbian custom to bring a gift when visiting, but I had barely managed to find a gift, a box of biscuits, in the one store that was open.

The evening before our planned departure, the Sniper advised me to cancel the trip. He told me it was a set-up. There was going to be a clash between local mafia gangs that were composed of both Croats and Serbs. Dr. Dario, whose best friend had been killed in one such ambush at the beginning of war, was on their hit list. I was terrified, of course, but I had to do something to avoid more bloodshed. I went to see Dario and we had a cup of coffee. I often read the grounds in my colleagues' coffee cups for the fun of it to tell them their fortunes. I told Dr. Dario that we weren't going to take the trip because I saw a coffin in his cup. He understood what I was trying to say, so we didn't go. The next day, we heard that someone had attacked a car that looked like the one that we were going to use to travel to Perna. No one was killed, but the car was destroyed.

The next morning, Dr. Dario looked probingly into my eyes, then he tapped my shoulder and said: "This time he saved our asses!"

We never spoke of it again.

17. How Do We Tell the World
about the Reality We're Living in?

Jovan, who hails from Niš in southern Serbia, chides me about meeting the Sniper.

"He's crazy. He's as dangerous to himself as he is to anyone who get in his way. Why pay any attention to him at all? Get rid of that guy!"

"You're right," I answer. "But I look at it differently. Why is he in this situation? He needs help, and he's going to be a handful for any therapist who takes on his case."

I keep the information I get from the Sniper confidential — but I can't trust him, either. I simply can't trust anyone here ... not a soul.

Jovan stimulates our social life with his unique brand of merriment. He makes a casual remark about how we can go take a look at the shipment of medicine that just arrived in Kordun the day before to see whether there is anything we need. So, we go and if we find something we need, then we help ourselves to it even though it hasn't been offered. Jovan wants to change the way medicine is being shared between hospitals. Gradually, I'm beginning to understand him — as the saying goes, little strokes fell great oaks. Nothing can be done quickly. I now understand why he spoke to me about the Sniper. Yes, he does want to protect me from stress and pain, but more importantly, he needs me as an anesthesiologist.

He also cares enough to take the time (unofficially, of course) to create a congenial environment. He gives tempo, atmosphere, and color to the hospital. During these tense and boring evenings that we spend in isolation, he invites us to gatherings where he involves us in different activities. He'll produce a pack of cards and make a good-natured taunt: "Okay, who's ready to lose some money tonight? Who's got the guts to take me on?"

Sometimes he encourages us to sing.

"Poetry has kept our people alive, so we owe it a profound debt of gratitude. We were oppressed by the Turks for five centuries; then we were oppressed by Fascists for a decade; and then the Communists made our lives miserable for more than fifty years. We survived it all. And the Serbian people could not have survived tyranny without poetry. So, we're going to survive by singing. Let me hear you now!"

At other times, he offers his opinions.

"*To be or not to be, that is* not *the question.* Shakespeare got it wrong. He didn't know Serbs. They're treating us like a flock of sheep. The right question to ask is: *Where are we going to end up?* My dear Mr. Shakespeare, that ought to have been the question. Something is rotten in Yugoslavia — not Denmark — Yugoslavia … and in the world, generally speaking."

He's a superb accordion player. He can play a dance tune or a dirge with equal passion. He can make the accordion cry.

He has two daughters and a wife back in Niš. His girls play an upright piano for him over the telephone, and even at this distance he isn't overlooking their mistakes: "Ah, a mistake again, my dear. Two. That's a lot," he gently says. "You'll have to practice some more before Dad gets home!"

His harmonious relationship with his daughters brings peace to us all. After most of our group leaves Glina to return home, he alone stays with me. He gives me courage, even though I sometimes don't see him for two or three days in a row because we're both so busy. Although he's older than me, he isn't old enough to be my father, yet he still looks out for me as if he were a concerned parent.

"Why's our gal so glum today? How about chess or friendly game of cards?" Jovan would say with a smile. He's always pulling faces and making people laugh just as Draguljce, the Yugoslav cartoon character, does. It's his way of distracting you from the gravity concealed in his words and actions.

We often chat as we play chess or cards, so I become relaxed. One evening, I venture to read him passages from my diary. It's not going to be a private affair because other people are in the room. I'm shaken to discover that I'm unable to control my voice or hold back the tears. I sense the staff stopping to listen. After I finish reading, the dead silence is punctuated by sniffling, tears, and sobbing.

Jovan, instead, whistles and applauds enthusiastically.

"That's it! I felt you had something in you all along, but I wasn't able to put my finger on it. Now I know what it is. People of Banija, we have a Serbian Hemingway! Type it up — there's gotta be some clean bond typing paper around here — but you've gotta polish it up a bit. Cut all the philosophizing. Life's a greater philosopher than you are. Delete the generalizations. Then let me take another look at it."

"Why do you need to take another look at it?" I ask, surprised.

"You'll see. From now on, I'll be taking you to meet some interesting people around here. Write down everything you hear. It'll mean a lot to them one day. This is our history. This is a gift from someone greater than all of us. It doesn't belong solely to you and it shouldn't remain a secret. You have to tell this story — even if it means risking your personal safety — so people can hear it far and wide," he says, teasing me with a laugh.

I take him seriously, so I approach my task as a chronicler with more responsibility. There's no writing paper, so the back of discharge notes becomes my medium. There's no carbon paper, so I have to type each copy separately. I send these texts to publications, including *Srpski glas* and *Politika*.

I telephone home. I haven't seen my children in nearly three months. Marija is in school. She has to take a written exam in Serbian composition, so she's asking me how to structure her essay. I gave her some suggestions, but she still ends up getting a

C. That's the first time she's ever gotten a C. She's a straight-A student who won awards at regional competitions in Literature, Geography, and Chemistry. Now she's crying.

I want to comfort her but all I can say was this: "Be quiet, you little fool! You'll improve your grade. Do you know how many children here would be happy if the only reason they had to cry was a C? Not even the schools are functioning properly in Krajina anymore. I hope you never have any reason in life to cry about anything except for your grades!"

"Are you scolding me?" she asks.

"Of course not, darling. I'd love nothing more than to give you a hug," I reply.

Ljuba is almost six years old! Her birthday is coming up. And I'm so far away.

"We went sledding yesterday. Grandpa Zlatan took us. The Fortress is covered with snow. But we ended up freezing. Grandpa said that it's even colder for you and those kids over there. I didn't want to cry, but my fingers were turning blue from the cold even though I had gloves on. Mom, am I Serbian like those children in Krajina?"

"Yes, just like the children in Krajina," I reply. "Why do you ask?"

I'm surprised by the changes I see in her. She's still a young child, after all.

"I'd like to help them. *The Serbs should be united.* That's what Grandpa said. Do you treat children?

"Yes, my child, I treat children, as well."

"Like me?"

"Just like you!"

"God Bless you, Mom! May the Army protect you! And when you come home, save one child and bring it here so that we can take care of it, so we can play together."

I put down the receiver and burst into tears.

Dara's Story

I'm not the only one who left children at home. Dr. Dara Pa-jić, the young anesthesiologist who's my friend and roommate, hasn't see her son Dino for a whole year. She's not crying about it.

She was born in Serbia, and had married a man from Kordun named Đuro while she was still at university. They are happily married and are very attached to each other. Their occasional embraces are passionate. They live in Tušilović, a suburb of Kar-lovac, in Croatia. They told me about the scare tactics the Croa-tian MUP (*i.e.*, the security services) used to put pressure on Serbs. The war began there long before the Serbian media began paying any attention to it. Dara and her husband quietly thought everything through. Then they decided to organize a resistance movement. They found a way to sneak out of the village and go into the mountains. Dara, a slender, fragile woman, often kept guard. Then the war began. Đuro was mobilized by the Serbian Army, and was later promoted to battalion commander; Dara was first sent to Vojnić and then to Vrgin Most where she served as a doctor.

Dara's mother- and father-in-law are on the front line on the other side of Korana, which is under attack by snipers. But they didn't want to leave the area. They were born there and don't care if they are killed. They didn't want to live out their old age in a refugee camp. They have land, personal property, and live-stock, which is their livelihood. Đuro is eighty kilometers away; Dara one hundred. Their son, Dino, who's still a boy, was sent to her mother's house in Čačak, Serbia.

Later during the war, she was transferred to Glina and then to the VMA, where she was supposed to take a course in anesthesi-ology because there were no anesthesiologists in Glina. So she packed her suitcase again and ventured into the unknown. But she ended up staying in Belgrade for less than a month and a half. Krajina wasn't a part of Yugoslavia any more, while the VMA in Belgrade was still considered Yugoslav territory. The chaos and the ensuing obstacles quickly multiplied according to the emerging political realities of a country that had, until recently, been united. No one wanted to pay for her specialization.

She arrived in Glina a week before I did. Dragica, our first Nurse Anesthetist, told me after we had gotten to know each other better: "Doctor Mitić, I'm looking forward to working with you. And I'm even happier that Dara will finally have a real teacher. She arrived seven days ago and she has already lost ten kilos. She is very responsible, but this work is, after all, for experienced doctors and not for beginners."

Dara arrived after having spent a weekend in Tušilović. They put her up in my room in the Department of Internal Medicine. It was a hospital room with three beds. I shied away from rooming with another woman because I have few women friends. I realized long ago that I could create the impression of being stand-offish. I simply don't like chatting endlessly about trivialities as young women generally do. I don't have the personality to engage in such conversations because they exhaust me. I'm quickly bored by complaints about husbands and mothers-in-law. When my anger boils over, I take action. Fortunately, it turned out that Dara shares my disposition.

She was lucky to have met Đuro — they're a perfect pair. They are, above all, adaptable. They hurry home to see each other twice a month. Dara prepares herself days in advance. She may be melancholy and exhausted when she sets off on her journey, but when she returns, she's on cloud nine.

"I love him, Sarah," she says. "Đuro's a great guy. It's only because of him that I agreed to be far away from our son — I agreed to it because I love Đuro."

As she speaks, she walks around the room in her silk underwear. She's unaffected, graceful, lovable, elegant, and lively.

I've always been certain that real love possesses a radiant quality, and knowing her is all the proof I need.

"Dara, why don't you go somewhere safe? You're in the middle of nowhere out here. Where will you go if Đuro gets killed?"

"While he's here, I belong to him. I've been with these people for nine years already even though I don't have legal status here. I'd be ashamed to leave now. The Medical Board sends me on different assignments as they see fit. They don't even ask me if I'm capable of doing everything they assign me to do. But I keep trying! I can't abandon Đuro. As long as he's here, I'm here too."

"You see Đuro so little. How do you cope?" I ask her.

"How?" she asks, looking surprised. "Well, we manage. I love him. I don't ask for anything else. I suppose he does everything other men do when they're far away from their wives or lonely. I'm neither a fool nor narrow-minded. But he's mine, and he often tells me: *Daruska, do whatever you want to do. It's war. Who knows if we'll still be alive tomorrow?*"

We sit with our legs crossed on our uncomfortable beds. She gesticulates as she talks. I absorb her every word and catch the nuances of her expression. She's a waterfall of life.

"O, look!" I said once, when I was reading the coffee grounds at the bottom of her cup. "Đuro's at the door!"

I was joking, of course, but just two hours later, there was a mighty banging on our door. We shouted that the visitor was free to enter. Then a giant of a man entered the room, a smile beaming on his face.

Dara jumped out of bed.

"O Đuro, you're here!" she cried in disbelief. "Sarah, you must be psychic! Đuro, Sarah predicted that you were going to come less than two hours ago!"

They're a funny pair because they resemble an elephant and a mouse. Đuro is a huge man, tall and bulky, while Dara is a delicate woman who barely reaches his armpit when she stands next to him. She disappears into his arms in the blink of an eye.

Đuro is an exceptional man. He invited me one day to join him and Dara for lunch. He understood the anxious glint in my eyes.

"Yes, we're in the Pink Zone (*i.e.*, the UN Protected Zone), but we're still alive," he assured me.

Two weeks later, a group of us went to visit Đuro's family home. Marko and Dara also became good friends. Every time Marko came to the hospital to visit me, Dara left the room and offered him her chair. She was that kind of friend. Marko and Đuro already knew each other. His parents welcomed us like family. A lamb and a piglet were roasting on a spit, and for me, the vegetarian, there were plenty of vegetables. Standing in stark contrast to the festive atmosphere, the windows of the house were taped over so that glass shattering because of nearby explosions wouldn't then injure people indoors.

As Đuro was showing us around his parents' home, a shot rang out in the neighborhood, and then the sounds of wailing. Đuro and Marko ran out and disappeared behind the house.

They quickly returned and explained that a soldier, who was guarding a bridge that separated the warring areas of Croatia from those of the Republic of Krajina, had been strangled. He was young. We were hearing the loud wailing of his parents and relatives. They brought the body to his family's home. The young man's face was contorted and his complexion was now dark blue, like that of a hanged man. He was on guard duty with an older, more experienced soldier who had passed out of sight, while the younger man remained standing guard in front of a family home. The attacker had lowered himself down from the roof and grabbed hold of the strap of the young man's field glasses, and he strangled him with it. He hadn't struggled much. It was over in two minutes.

All this had happened before dawn. His older friend, who had no walkie-talkie or cell phone, didn't come back to the front of the house to look for him until morning. Now he was in agony. He was drunk. He wouldn't allow anyone to approach him. He had been a close friend of the young man. The bridge was only about fifty meters from Ðuro and Dara's house. The thought that some-one could come on any given night and strangle a guard or mem-bers of a family made my flesh crawl. Yet there hadn't been any such killings until now. Things are getting even more dangerous. The Croats are escalating their attacks. They're up to something.

I tried to orient myself to reality: *I am in Ðuro's parents' home, which is filled with the sounds of wailing. This is the bru-tal reality of our lives.*

I keep repeating to myself: *It's 1993. Spring is coming. I'm a doctor, a volunteer in the Republic of Serbian Krajina, a self-proclaimed state of Serbian rebels who rose up against the Croatian government that had seceded from Yugoslavia and thereby denied Serbs the status of equal citizens. I am in love with Colonel Marko Vrcelj, the Glina Commander. I am in love with the struggle of the Serbian people to survive and to keep their centuries old territories. In Serbia, 800 km away, I have two children who are waiting for me to come back home. There's no reason for me to expect a welcoming committee in Serbia, aside from my children and parents. The Republic of Serbian Krajina is an unwelcome problem for Serbs in Serbia as well as for Serbian President Slobodan Milošević.*

The mere thought of the situation in Krajina causes the Serbs, as well as their leader, anguish. The unemployment rate in Kraj-ina is incredibly high — out of 430,000 Serbs, only 36,000 of them are employed. Industry, agriculture, and anything that could be considered economically productive or that could foster any kind of economic security has been destroyed. Krajina is entirely made up of illusion and improvisation. The Communist state controlled all the institutions as well as their financing, but nothing is functioning now and no one knows who's in charge. The newly declared Republic of Krajina stands no chance of survival without help from Serbia.

Serbs are fighting for the survival of Yugoslavia, but the International Community keeps insisting that they are fighting for "Greater Serbia." The International Community took the side of the Croats and it doesn't support the Serbs, who are simply fighting for their rights. These Serbs were born here and the Serbian people have been living here for five centuries. Where are they going to go now? The sadness is overwhelming. The Serbs have no future in Krajina because Serbia is not lending them support.

The International Community is arming Croatia. Retired U.S. generals are joining the conflict on the side of the Croats; and they are drawing up the Croatian Army's battle plans. The Serbs in Krajina are, for the most part, civilians who have no prior military experience. Only 30,000 of them are actually capable of carrying a weapon. Volunteers from Serbia who have no experience, who are disorganized, and who are hard to deal with are the only ones who came to help. The people of Krajina would be better off without their support because these volunteers only added to the criminal activity going on in Krajina. Out of some two thousand such volunteers, Marko could only sign on about a hundred.

The authorities in Krajina are semi-literate puppets who are being controlled by the regime in Serbia, which has no idea of what is really going on here. The only thing I am one-hundred percent certain of is that I hate politics. I hate politicians. All of them!

We just lost Blinski Kut — a part of Krajina close to Glina. Jovan kept saying that I was not in Krajina simply to discharge my duties as a doctor — to care for the sick and wounded —

because destiny has given me an additional task: to record local history.

Jovan lived up to his word. Whenever there's time, he takes me to meet people. Their stories are authentic testimonies of the atrocities of war. On this particular day, we visited the father of Dragiša Stefanović, who was the very first victim of the war in Glina.

Another Family Story

Two graves, a wreath, and a cross stand before a house near a filling station on the road to Petrinja.

On June 26, 1991, the day after Croatia declared independence, the Ministry of Internal Affairs (MUP) of Croatia attacked the mostly Serbian area of Glina. About 1,200 well-armed Croatian paramilitaries set out from Petrinja in central Croatia for Glina, about nineteen kilometers away.

In Glina, about 500 men were supposedly ready to fight, but as so often happens during civil wars — especially brother fighting brother over land they've shared for centuries, which weakens moral resolve — most of them had a change of heart, so they deserted. Only fifty of the bravest men remained. One of these young men was Dragiša Stefanović. After he had launched his last grenade, he was shot in the back by a Croat from the attic window of a nearby house. The gunman was his neighbor.

Jovan introduces me to Dragiša's father. The old man takes us to the neighbor's attic to see the bullet holes. The mere sight of the place sends a chill down my spine. We go up a narrow stairway that's lined with plastic bags full of trash. We enter that miserable attic where old clothes lay scattered on the floor. The windowsill and walls have been ripped up by gunfire from automatic weapons.

Then Dragiša's father brings out a photo album. In each picture, we see a handsome, well-built young man smiling happily. In several photographs, he's wearing a white *jujitsu* outfit. He had a black belt and was a member of the national team. His father holds the album, and absentmindedly relates details from the young man's life. *He never drank, never smoked, he never ...* the old man mumbles on as though he's wondering how the boy could have perished.

Another photograph shows a women's detachment that was formed by Dragiša's father after he returned from imprisonment in Croatia. One young woman's face mingles a winsome smile with the distracted look of a poet. Her name was Rajka. She and her brother were children of a mixed marriage. Her brother stayed in Sisak, where he was drafted into the Croatian National Guard (ZNG), while Rajka became a dominant force in the Glina Women's Regiment.

She had written on the photo: "O, when will this war end, so brother and sister can be together again?"

It was early evening when Rajka was killed. She used the wrong password. Rifle fire cut her down and soon she was lying dead with her eyes open. When the guard saw his reflection in her eyes, he nearly killed himself. Later, her brother was killed as well. The two graves near the filling station are theirs.

There's no more room in my mind for new misfortunes. I lean on Jovan and begin crying. I just can't take anymore.

"Sarah ... all this is life," says Jovan. "One bullet erases the past as well as the future."

We hurry down the main street. On the left, we pass a marble and glass memorial. It was built in memory of some 1,500 men, women, and children from Banija who had been massacred in the old Serbian church at the beginning of World War II.

An old man from Glina, who survived that mass killing, related this story to us the other day:

"For days, armed Croatian Ustaše were driving local Serbs into the church. None of us knew what was awaiting us. The executioners relentlessly slaughtered their victims. Even beasts have a more benign expression on their faces when they're tearing their prey to pieces than these Ustaše killers had. The victims refused to show any sign of fear to those devils. That was their only retaliation. They died silently. Their life blood flowed from their slit throats onto the floor and then drained into the street. New groups of victims had to wade through the blood, ankle-deep. Neither wailing nor cries for mercy could be heard — not a single one. It was protest by death."

After the war, the church was demolished and a Memorial Center was built in its place, but the Communists amply demonstrated their contempt by placing the toilets on the very spot where the altar once stood. The Communists introduced drastic changes to cast the memory of these killings into oblivion. Today, ownership of this Memorial has reverted to the Serbian Orthodox Church.

Serbian history is cyclical.

"Our children were born from that blood and from those memories," the old man defiantly said. "Serbs, beware of Croats! Those devils appease themselves only temporarily with blood."

A Young Mother Tries to Commit Suicide

The cold air helps me shake off the dire impressions these stories have left. Jovan becomes self-absorbed. He lifts his head, pulls up the collar of his coat, and gazes in the distance. Along the way, an ambulance pulls up alongside us.

The driver opens the door and shouts: "They're waiting for you, Doc! A gunshot victim — a woman tried to kill herself."

We jump into the ambulance. The memories of slaughter and the meditations on death vanish. My tears stop. I turn back into a doctor once again. After we arrive, I run to the dressing station. On the table, I see a young woman who's about twenty years old. She's pale. Her eyes are shut, but she's breathing normally. As I put on my scrubs, the nurses removed her torn and soiled blouse.

She had shot herself at close range. Her huge breasts, trembling uncontrollably, are swollen with milk that's flowing from them.

The woman is unresponsive, so she can't answer any questions.

"Where's the baby?" I ask right away.

"They took it to the maternity ward," says a nurse.

The wound looks terrible. The bullet had passed through the stomach and exited under the left breast. She was lucky. Her blood pressure and pulse are normal, but she's pale from shock. I anesthetize her without having any data about her. A urologist from Zemun speaks up:

"She's my patient. It's a flesh wound. I'll perform the surgery."

He operates on her. He's right. Her belly fat and her clumsiness with the weapon — and perhaps her wish to go on living, after all — saved her. As she regains consciousness, Nurse Ljiljana and I hold her hand. We wait for her to open her eyes. We're patient. I press her face lightly from time to time.

In the meanwhile, I informed myself about her case. She was a *primipara*, a woman who was giving birth to her first child. It had been an uneventful pregnancy and she delivered at term. The Maternity Ward advised me that she had been discharged three days ago without any apparent complications. She lives in a village twenty kilometers from Glina. Her mother-in-law came to bring her home from the hospital. Her husband is on the front lines. They have a daughter. The midwives say she had complained that she and her husband were poor. Their cow has just calved, so they can't milk her. The calf is sucking up all the milk. She's afraid that she won't have enough milk. She said that she didn't know anything about nursing a baby. The midwives explained everything to her. She seemed to look forward to every breast-feeding. She went home on foot with her aged mother-in-law because there's no transportation.

She and her mother-in-law have to do all the house work. There's no water, so they have to walk two kilometers to a well. And there's no electricity. They've used up all the propane, so they're waiting for her husband to return from the front in order to buy some more because they don't have any money. The two women are alone in the dark. The baby has only its mother's breast. There are no pacifiers, baby bottles, diapers, or visiting nurses. They were alone and scared with a crying baby. Whenever the baby begins to cry, its mother gave it her breast. She was squeezing milk into its small mouth. A second later, the baby choked and went blue. The inexperienced mother thought her baby was dead. She left the baby and took the gun that had been standing next to the door ever since the war began, and fired it, aiming straight for her heart. As fate would have it, her husband was just returning. When he heard the gunshot, he was already in the yard. He ran two kilometers to reach a neighbor who had a car and they brought her to the hospital unconscious with the baby. The baby girl was going to be all right. She was only dehydrated and hungry.

Nurse Ljiljana and I wait while the girl opens her eyes cautiously.

"How's my baby?" she asks.

"She's fine!" we say in unison.

"And what about me?"

"You are fine, too. Thanks more to luck than anything else."

She gazes at the ceiling, then she begins crying.

"It would have been better if I had died," she says. "I haven't got anything. How am I going to raise my daughter?"

Ljiljana embraces her.

"My son's eighteen months old. When I fled Sisak, I was in the same situation you're in now, maybe even worse. You've at least got your own house and some livestock. I didn't have a damn thing! I had two bags, some clothes, two small children, and a newborn son. I had no milk. Sometimes I wonder where I got the strength to keep moving, but I wasn't going to give up! I'm not going to die without putting up a fight. My neighbors found me a room, they took up a collection and got some rags and diapers, and they found a milk cow. My son's a growing boy. He's got six teeth now and he says *Mama... Mama*. I'll give you his left-over baby things, and we'll take up a collection for you. Why didn't you come to us for help?"

The woman sighs. She must have imagined her life and marriage differently at one time. The war has changed everything. She's silent for a moment, then she begins crying again.

I quietly leave the room. Ljiljana is her best company now. They understand each other. The next day, I transferred her to the Gynecology Ward. It's better to dress her wounds there than to bring the baby into the ICU, which is filthy.

Ordinary Nights

Snow fell but it melted only a few days later. I'm grateful that it isn't very cold. We have heating only when the emergency generator is working, and now we're running out of fuel oil. At night, oil lamps light the corridors so that our patients can at least find their way to the toilet. Desk lamps serve to light the nurses' rooms. The Hospital Director, who purchased the generator, figured out how to rig the cables to connect the ICU with the Nurse's Room in the Surgical Ward so they wouldn't be in complete darkness at night. Sometimes it's the only light we've got in the OR during surgery. We have to aim two flickering flashlights at the patient whenever we have batteries.

Once, during a bombardment, I ran straight into a Croat commando who had broken into the hospital. We wouldn't have discovered him unless a soldier and I had gone up the darkened staircase to his room in the attic to find some flashlights he had in his duffle bag. I'll never forget being startled by the ominous shadow of a camouflaged figure aiming a gun straight at me with its outstretched arm. I could see a silencer at the end of the barrel. I was paralyzed by fear. I couldn't even scream. Shock caused blood from the spontaneous rupture of capillaries to fill my throat. My ears went deaf. I wasn't even able to hear the orders the soldier accompanying me was shouting, even though he was right behind me. He shoved me down the staircase and he followed close behind. We got back up on our feet at the first landing and ran without looking back. We burst into the ICU, where we informed the guards of the intruder.

It turned out that there were several commandoes who were immediately apprehended. They had parachuted onto the slopes of Mt. Strmica. Someone from Knin was waiting for them there. The population is mixed, just as the hospital staff is, so it's difficult to know who's on which side. The commandoes walked right into the hospital unchallenged, just as when I had first come. There is practically no security at all because there is no clear enemy. The hospital guards found a trailer full of explosives outside that would surely have blown us all to smithereens if we hadn't stumbled upon the intruders.

I repressed this episode from my conscious mind, so I had completely forgotten it. But my body still remembers that horrible incident and to this very day I don't dare climb stairs alone at night in the dark. I always suspect that I may find someone pointing a gun at me on the next landing. To this day, I still can't figure out why those commandoes hadn't shot us. Maybe they were momentarily confused because they found themselves face to face with a woman. But they were planning to blow us all up to Kingdom Come. They would have killed women and children, too. I can't comprehend that. I'm still grateful that they didn't shoot me dead. The soldier I was with skillfully took advantage of their hesitation and saved our lives, but these memories still come back to haunt me on every dark staircase.

These memories are vile. I'll never escape them. I can't call them out into the open daylight and fight them as if they were physical beings, and vanquish them once and for all. I'm never free of these phantoms. When I came here, I wasn't even afraid of the bullets. Now I'm afraid of the dark as if I were a child. I ask the nurses to see me to my room. They understand because they too have experienced emotional trauma, so they aren't going to make fun of me. On the contrary, they're considerate. Whenever they need to come and wake me up for a surgical intervention, they wait for me in my room with a small lamp. I always get up quickly because I sleep in my clothes. I miss feeling the sheets on my bare legs.

I see headlight beams moving along the walls of my darkened room. An ambulance is arriving. The elevator isn't working, so they have to carry the patients on a stretcher up the stairs to the hospital beds. One young man, his face flushed and dripping with sweat, is lying on one stretcher. A medical nurse in military fatigues is accompanying him. She appears to be as small and as frail as a child. At first, I think it's a boy. Her eyes are large and serious. She stands at attention and reports to me. We remove the man's shirt, and while I auscultate his breathing and heartbeat, I look furtively at the tiny soldier. She's so thin that I wonder how she can endure the front lines. Her name is Nada. She's the only female paramedic. All the other paramedics are men. She has to sleep on a stretcher because there aren't any beds. It's amazing what women are capable of doing. It's hard enough in peacetime; but during war, it's a hundred times worse.

"I think he suffered a heart attack," says Nada. "It started suddenly. He was suffocating. He could hardly breathe."

I took his EKG.

"He didn't have a heart attack, Nada," I reply. "Judging from his symptoms, I think he has pneumonia. I'll take a chest X-ray tomorrow. I don't want to wake up the radiologist."

"Am I free to go now?" she asks brusquely.

"Of course, you are. Rest up a bit first. Go get something to eat in the kitchen downstairs," I say.

"Thank you, but I'm still on duty. I have to go back to Petrinja."

Nada marches off. She has performed her duty, but something about this girl puts me ill at ease. Who wiped the smile off her face? Who made her put on a uniform instead of a dress? Who made a soldier out of her? These unpleasant thoughts disturb me, so I can't fall asleep for a long time. The bed keeps creaking as I toss and turn.

Young Men Crippled for Life

Dead men keep passing through my hands until they stink of death. I wash my hands a hundred times a day. I shower whenever I can, but the smell isn't just coming from my hands — it's emanating from the very air around me. Some are brought in dead; others die right before my eyes. There are many occasions when we doctors have to go to the waiting room and break the bad news to loved ones: *You have my deepest sympathy.*

The first time I had to do this was back in 1991 during the war in Knin. As a doctor in Serbia, I also had to do it on occasion, but as an anesthesiologist I was less likely to be called upon. Uncontrollable weeping and wailing inevitably followed my expression of sympathy. Some people fainted; others cursed. But in Glina, it surprises me to see that they just stare back at me in silence. They nod their heads as if I were vanishing from their sight. An agonizing sigh follows. They hold their heads, then crouch down slowly against a wall. It's as if they want to become smaller so the news would hurt less. They sigh deeply a few times, then abruptly stand up and straighten their posture. They shake my hand. Then they immediately become matter of fact and ask: *When can we claim the body?* There are no tears, no howls of anguish, because death is an everyday occurrence.

That was why I was surprised to hear frightful screams coming from a corridor in the Surgical Department. At first, there was a crash. Then a terrible howl followed. Finally, screaming. I ran out into the corridor and what I saw immediately caused my adrenalin to kick in. A patient was lying under an overturned wheelchair. He was a wounded soldier whose lower legs had been amputated. He was lying in a pool of urine, and a little further away I saw his bedpan, which he had cast aside. Pain distorted his features. He was, otherwise, a handsome young man, but now he looked dreadful. His teeth were clenched, and he was snarling like a wounded animal. Nurse Dušanka, whom we called Duda, was bent over him and quietly weeping.

"Get the fuck out of here!" he screams.

"Calm down," Duda whispers.

"What's the fucking use? Am I going to feel any better? Damn straight I'm not. None of this shit's gonna do me any fuckin good. Fuck this wheelchair, and alla you can go fuck yourselves, too! I'm only twenty-five, and my legs are gone. I don't need your fuckin blubbering."

Duda began crying aloud. The other nurses were silent, petrified with fear. We all knew that he had the right to express his feelings of rage and frustration. He was angry with life, with his fate, with God. But prolonging the scene wasn't going to help anyone.

I stepped right up and took charge.

"Who's causing this racket?" I demand loudly. "You: why are you yelling at the top of your lungs like a spoiled brat?"

The patient looks at me astonished. He isn't expecting this.

"Get up!" I order.

I put up the wheelchair upright, set the brake, and then I fix my eyes on him.

"Come on, I'm going to hold it, and you get up on it."

"Are you kidding me?" he says. "I can't do that."

"Don't you try to fool me … I know damn well you can!"

"What do I hold onto?" he asks, looking at me as his rage turns to scorn. "What the fuck do you think you're doing, anyway? You're a fucking nut job!"

"You've got a strong pair of arms," I say, keeping my voice even. "What you can't do with your legs anymore, you have to do with your arms. You've got two strong arms but you're sniveling like a baby. I don't pity you. You're the one feeling sorry for yourself."

"Get the fuck outa my face!" he shouts, glaring at me with undisguised hostility.

"I'll show you how to do it ... watch me."

I sit on the floor beside him. Duda is holding the wheelchair. Resting on my hands, I drag myself slowly to the lowest part of the wheelchair and little by little, by supporting myself against the wheelchair, I manage to raise myself to the seat.

I break into a sweat. I stand up. I look at him furiously.

"Come on, it's going to be easier for you because you're stronger, and, forgive my saying so, your legs are shorter."

He's completely perplexed, but his eyes shine somehow. I provoked his competitive spirit. He makes up his mind to give it a try. He swings thrice with his hands and he's up in the wheelchair.

"I'm better than you are, Doc!" he says, grinning. "I'm going to change my clothes now. I pissed all over myself."

Duda ran after him, but he turned around and said with an impish smile: "Find me a younger nurse, Goca, for instance. She's a babe. Duda, comrade! I'm sorry, but you're too old for me!"

After this, I didn't go to see the patient for a day or so. I wanted to let him think things over. Two days later, when I happened to be in his room to see a patient who had just been operated on, he looked at me with a smile and said:

"Don't worry, he's breathing normally. He's awake. I'll look after him. I've seen a lot of patients like him over the past year. I've learned almost everything. You don't have to send Sandra."

Then he shifted his position in the wheelchair and skillfully opened a small cabinet.

"Here's something I want to give you," he said, and he took out a bottle with homemade fruit juice.

"Take it. It's made from our Muscat grapes. It's got a nice aroma. When I get the prostheses, I'll be able to cultivate our vineyards again. The physiotherapist said that I'll be able to do everything myself."

I took the fragrant fruit juice from him. Now we were comrades.

I winked at him: "Thank you, my friend. You're still better than I am!"

I took the bottle to my room and I opened it immediately. We couldn't buy fruit juice here. I hadn't tasted any fruit or juice for more than two months. The fact that he had decided to give me this valuable gift meant a great deal. His kind gesture strengthened my relationship with all the others. I began to feel accepted, and that my contributions were being recognized.

18. Springtime and Love

The Croats are attacking Glina again in an attempt to cut Krajina off from Serbia. We're already accustomed to these attacks, so we don't even give them a second thought, much less do we consider the possibility that the Croats might burst through the doors at any moment. *Let the things happen as they must*, is our philosophy.

One day during the siege, they brought in a wounded Croat soldier who was a JNA prisoner. He had a leg wound. A bullet had shattered his ankle-bone. He's thirty-three years old and he comes from a village near Sisak. Since our hospital is small, we accommodate him in a bed behind curtains because that's the only way of sequestering him. Two JNA soldiers keep watch over him. At first, he's silent, but then he starts talking to them. He's a woodcutter who has a wife and a child. He had been conscripted like many others.

The next day, we were going to reinforce his shattered foot with metal plates. We had enough material. Technician Velimir asked if we should perform the operation under local anesthesia to conserve anesthetics. No, I told him. We were going to operate under general anesthesia. Then it would be easier for him as well as for the medical team. Imagine what could happen if we had our usual problems during surgery. Would the patient think that it was bad luck or malicious intent? He might as well sleep through the operation. His patient history indicated that he had been taking opioids for the last few months — in order not to feel the cold, he told us. I anesthetized him normally, but later I saw that he needed larger doses of narcotics than were normally necessary. That was quite common among Croatian soldiers who were our patients.

After a few days, we went to see the patient. His foot looked fine.

"You didn't have to take so much trouble," he said.

"Why?" I asked him, surprised.

"Come on!" he said. "The food's all right. Your men share everything with me. We even got cake. When I was wounded and captured, I almost smiled. It sounds crazy, I know, but I was happy. I was captured by men who had — until recently — been my acquaintances. I knew everything would turn out okay. Why are we divided? We worked here together as our fathers did. I don't know why this has happened to us. All I know is that I'm safe now."

A commotion arose in the room. The other wounded soldiers were all agreeing with him. They'd had enough. They wanted peace.

Representatives from the Red Cross and UNPROFOR appeared shortly thereafter. I was surprised that they showed no interest in the wounded Serbian soldiers. They wanted to get in touch with this prisoner. In my own naïve fashion, I reported it to the JNA soldiers guarding the prisoner.

They stared at me coldly and answered sharply: "We have orders from the Commander that foreign citizens can see prisoners only with his written permission."

I immediately understood, and I was happy with the answer. I communicated this information to the Hospital Director and to the representatives of both organizations. The Director checked again on the phone, and then talked to the UNPROFOR commander. He translated everything into German for the newcomers. There wasn't a trace of regret in his voice. He was courteous and polite.

"He is, gentlemen, our prisoner of war. We're the national army. You may have access to his medical records, and you may see him — without verbal contact — from the corridor."

The UNPROFOR commander gave up trying to see the patient. They weren't interested in his condition, after all. All they were interested in was his testimony, which they would later use for their own purposes. I had suspected as much.

The Director asked them if they were just as eager to see wounded Serbian prisoners on the Croatian side. Yes, sometimes, the representative of the Red Cross replied, but he said someone else is in charge of that.

"Yes, I understand," the Director said. "That's God's department!"

We bade them farewell with cynical smiles. This time, thanks to the attitude of our Commander, we had managed to retain our dignity.

A little later, I went to the Commander and asked him why he had acted this way and whether he was afraid of the consequences.

"They're on our territory," he said. "It's protected by the regular army and whoever finds himself on our territory has to obey the rules — especially guests. They skillfully manipulate the prisoner, giving him moral support and promising to raise public awareness of his case that will lead to his release. That's how we lost many prisoners, as well as a lot of valuable information that we could have gotten out of enemy soldiers. UNPROFOR and the Red Cross are always trying to hamstring us, but we put an end to that. He's our prisoner of war and he is going to be treated according to the rules of the Geneva Convention."

The Geneva Convention states that international organizations must not be biased toward the wounded of any particular nationality. Even so, we witness precisely this type of bias every single day. They're only taking care of Muslims and Croats. They ignore wounded Serbs. The arrogance of UNPROFOR and the Red Cross is not only unconcealed but also insulting. After all, we're only human.

March is already gone and April is somersaulting in. I'm watching the gathering dusk through the windows of the first floor. The sky is turning orange between the Administration Building and the pine trees. Daffodils are springing up along the tree-lined promenade. Pigeons are cooing.

Spring is here!

I hope that spring isn't going to usher war into Serbia, too. In that case, we'd end up spending the rest of our lives overcoming the horror and despair of witnessing the destruction of our country. The war has already been going on for three years, and the people who remain here are tense and hypersensitive, so they fly off the handle easily. They are oppressed by uncertainty, yet they manage to carry on with their lives. They socialize, they fall in love, they have children. Life goes on with its promise of fulfillment and hope for the future. I find it strange at first, but later

I realize it's wonderful that love songs can be heard despite the roar of weaponry.

War, Epigenetics, and Me

A war takes place every generation in the Balkans. Some generations have even survived two wars in a single lifetime. These people have a higher tolerance for stress than people from other parts of the world do — those who don't share our history.

Epigenetics is the study of inherited experiences. I sometimes wondered about the source of my resilience in facing the many challenges I had come up against. After my stay in Krajina, I realized that my parents gave me this resilience to trauma because they had survived similar impossible situations. In addition to war, natural disasters and floods, earthquakes and tsunamis also give rise to such resilience. The stress experienced by large groups of people may be divided into six stages.

Stage I is a state of chaos characterized by intense fear, which is accompanied by temporarily disoriented thinking. Stage II is comprised of organizing and focusing on finding solutions in order to survive. This stage gives rise to intense anxiety, during which biological functions begin to fail and all of one's energy must be focused on survival. Stage III may be characterized as a honeymoon period, a time of reorganization which is distinguished by a zest for life. The actual situation cannot be properly assessed during this period of euphoria. During Stage III, the libido partially recovers. It's part of the euphoria, but it may also include a weakening of traditional sexual boundaries. Stage IV is an awakening during which people finally become fully aware of what had happened to them. Stage V is marked by depression and disappointment. The duration of this stage depends on the extent of individual suffering. Stage VI is a period of realignment, a time to search for new meaning in life and for new reasons to continue to fight for survival.

I understand that the people around me are experiencing Stage III collective shock and stress. They are happy to have survived the initial Croatian attacks, and they are now better organized, and they have found new meaning in their society. During this stage, they remain unaware of the fact that they are isolated and bereft of any political and/or legal prospects. They are surviving, which is all-important.

I too am swept up in their joy and optimism. Even so, my children are in Serbia and I know that it's unnatural for me to be separated from them for such a long period of time. My living reality is not exclusively positive. The inevitable question arises: *What is going to happen to us after this euphoric stage is over?*

Jagoda and Igor

Jagoda, one of our nurses, and Igor, a surgeon, met during the liberation of Koštajnica from Croatian paramilitaries. She was widowed before the war began. She has two girls. She's young, raven-haired, and green–eyed. She's a passionate and dedicated nurse. One day, not long after the war began, they brought in ten corpses to the Outpatient Department at the Koštajnica Medical Center, where she was working. These were the bodies of young men whom she recognized as her neighbors.

"I worked like a robot," she told me. "I wasn't even aware of the fact that they were all dead. I saw the bullets wounds, and their bodies were still warm as if they were still alive. I felt somehow intimate with them. I didn't want to admit to myself that they were dead. The next day, black flags covered the street. My neighbors were wearing black scarves. Death was everywhere. It finally dawned on me that my friends and acquaintances were dead and gone. Everything had changed. I had changed, too. I left the Outpatient Department and volunteered for combat duty with the JNA. They were going to need me. I triaged the wounded, dressed their wounds, and prepared them for transport. I encouraged them. They felt braver in the presence of a woman."

It was there, while she was hunched over a wounded soldier to whom she was giving first aid under sniper fire, that she locked horns with one of the soldiers.

"Get out of here!" he barked.

"Go to hell!" she shot back. "I'm a nurse!"

"That's cute, Nurse. Your gotta head as hard as Bosnian granite!" the soldier angrily retorted. "Please allow me to introduce myself. I'm Dr. Igor!"

And that was how they first met. A year and a half later, they're still seeing each other.

Jagoda is living in a small Bosnian town where she's working in a health center. She's also looking after her mother as well as her two children. Igor is moving around the front lines. He has no permanent assignment. His wife left him and went to Germany because the war was too much for her to bear. Igor was trying to heal the lingering emotional wounds that followed the end of his marriage. He, therefore, came to believe that both love and loyalty were most clearly revealed in times of trials and great difficulties. Even though he felt deceived and abandoned, he was still alive and his soul remained intact. When Igor and Jagoda met, love pierced their hearts more quickly than any bullet ever could have. After they exchanged glances and touched each other's hands, the war took on a new color. He's honest, dedicated, and responsible. They can't enjoy each other's company whenever they wish, but they cope with the difficulties and they make do with what they've got.

One night, Igor came to the hospital; Jagoda arrived half an hour later. She had to drive fifty kilometers alone at night. One stretch of the road was under constant sniper fire.

"I drove five kilometers, blind, through the dark without any lights. That's how I solved the sniper problem," she laughed.

"And it's worth it because I love him! That's all that's left after material things vanish: Love!"

Her eyes were glowing with inner light. I believed her, and I envied her.

Their problem was finding a place to stay. Dara had gone to see Đuro in Tušilović, so I was alone. I let them use my room. I would then sleep in the ICU, where there was a free bed. I screened off my bed by the window from the adjacent patient, and I lay down. It happened to be the only unoccupied bed in the wing. In the morning, I laughed heartily when I saw that Igor had given Jagoda pine cones, which he had brought from the mountains, as earrings. The weekend passed quickly. Over the past few days, snow has been falling unexpectedly, but it melts quickly so the roads are clear. Jagoda has to go back. God is gracious to lovers. The war destroyed their relationships, but it gave them new ones. Love lifts them above harsh reality and gives meaning to their desperation.

After they leave, I begin straightening up the room. That's when I find a crumpled piece of paper — it's a poem in Jagoda's handwriting:

> I gather kisses from your shoulders
> I string them on a chain of memories.
> I love you with my teeth clenched
> With a wordless tongue and trembling thighs,
> From passion felt but unexplained.
> I love you now for this moment.
> I know! There's no tomorrow!
> You ask me:
> What do you want?
> I remain silent, I have no aspirations.
> I enjoy being with you
> Today,

For today.
Tomorrow might not exist.
I gather my kisses from your shoulders
I string them on a chain of memories,
Memories.

Dr. Dario calls me into his office later that day. It's serious, so he's looking me straight in the eye. He says he's received complaints about my conduct. That's all I need! I'm caught off-guard. What kind of complaint can this be? Whom had I offended?

Dr. Dario claims that a nurse has filed a complaint about my having lent my room to people with "loose morals." The people in question were, of course, Jagoda and Igor. Jagoda was a beautiful blonde. The nurse who filed the complaint is a lady I seldom see. She suffers from morbid obesity and must weigh nearly 500 lbs. She's barely able to move. The chairs in the hospital can't hold her, so she had to have a chair specially made for her office.

It's strange that this person happened to be the one who found out what Jagoda and Igor were up to in my room, but I can't allow myself the luxury of laughing in Dario's face as he's telling me the story.

"What exactly did she say: *Immorality*? I bet she'd give all five hundred pounds of herself for a little taste of immorality. This is preposterous!"

Dario can't keep a straight face any longer.

"I caught her peeking through the keyhole," he confesses. "You should have seen it! I caught her red-handed, so she, of course, is going to blame someone else. You did let them stay in your room, after all!"

Our laughter shakes the room. It's not at all nice but we can't help it. Imagining the scene was hilarious: picture this nurse blocking the hallway with her super-sized *derrière* as she's peeking through the keyhole at Igor and Jagoda locked in a passionate embrace. *O la la!*

As our laughter subsides, I wonder: What's going to become of her? This nurse was forced to stay in Glina because she was too big to evacuate. She can't get through the doors of a car or a bus. They'd have to get an open trailer and hitch it to the back of a truck or bus. The very thought of it saddens me. How is she going to feel if she has to be left behind? How will she feel?

Glina's Hairdresser

When a woman starts feeling depressed, she usually changes her hairstyle or buys a new dress. I can't buy a dress here — or anything else, for that matter — but I can at least change my hairdo. Boba from Karlovac, a well-known hairdresser, has a salon in Topusko. He was exempted from active duty to set up a beauty school. The reasoning was that it would be good for morale to give women work and to let them help each other look attractive. Boba got a one-room apartment in Topusko, which he repurposed into a hair salon. In the morning, he holds classes; afternoons, he sees clients. He lives with his mother and six-year-old son. The boy's mother is Croatian; Boba is Serbian. He took the boy from his mother so now he's afraid she's going to have him kidnapped because she has clandestine connections with Croatian paramilitaries. Even though there's a border now, it's neither a reliable nor permanent boundary. Boba doesn't let his son out of his sight.

Over the past two months, my hair has gone limp and its color has faded. Nurse Dragica went to Topusko the other day and came back with a perfect new hairdo. She took a military vehicle there and hitchhiked back. Dara is a regular client. So Dara and I call the Director and tell him that we need a little R&R. Not only is he willing to grant us leave, but he also has an ambulance take us. We leave for Topusko immediately after our shift is over, but we still have to be back as soon as possible.

We drive the fifteen kilometers to Topuško. All the while, we're looking forward to Boba taking us because Dara helped him get his business started.

Boba is smartly dressed for a man swept up in a war. He's wearing a silk shirt, a fashionable necktie with a floral pattern, and Italian-made shoes. The only thing missing is a gold chain around his neck, as I'd seen Mile Paspalj, the shady politician from Krajina, wearing. Boba gives us the once-over and says in a dismissive tone that he can't fit us into his schedule. We have money, we said, but he still refused. His reason? He has no time! Dara begs him but our pleas fall on deaf ears, even after Dara reminds him that he owes her and Đuro for the life on Easy Street he's now enjoying. He says that he's exhausted — that women are nags — and ungrateful creatures.

Now I become self-conscious about my mud-spattered combat boots, my grimy jeans, and my bulky jumper. Should I have worn a nice silk dress? Should I have gone to another hairdresser beforehand to freshen up? Perhaps then he would have agreed to do my hair.

"She came all the way from Serbia!" Dara pleads. "She's risking her life to help people here, and you're refusing to do her hair — even if she pays for it?"

"No one's going to feel grateful for *that*!" he answers coldly.

As we're bickering, two girls accompanied by UNPROFOR soldiers stroll in. They don't have an appointment either, but they've got dollars, because ladies who entertain foreign soldiers get paid cash in dollars. Boba gives them a warm welcome while he gives us the brush off without so much as a word of apology. It's difficult to discern his priorities: is it the girls or the dollars?

A small blond boy runs into the room. Then he retreats shyly. I think of Ljuba, my younger daughter. I take out some coins and gave them to the boy. I tell him to buy himself a chocolate bar. The boy doesn't want to take it, so he lets the coins fall to the floor. Boba, though, bends over and pockets the loose change just as if I weren't there!

An expression of disbelief transfixes Dara's face. We say good-bye and then step into a fine drizzle outside. The soft light is turning everything grey.... We come upon UNPROFOR soldiers who won't let us take a paved road that goes past a school yard, so Dara and I grumpily slosh through open ground riddled with mud puddles. We don't know with whom to be angrier, the sycophantic hairdresser or the UNPROFOR soldiers who made him the man he is today. It'll be one happy day when those bastards turn their backs to leave. And I hope the door knob hits them in the ass on their way out!

The ambulance is coming to pick us up at 4:00 p.m. but it's only 1:30 p.m., so we head for the main road. At the railway switch, we see a weeping willow whose resplendent yellow branches are in full bloom with delicate flowers. My anger vanishes at the sudden sight of unexpected beauty. I wasn't going to let a bad-hair day spoil everything, no matter what.

There are some violets near the roadside. On the other side, yellow primroses are hiding in the underbrush.

"Look, Dara! The lake!" I say, trying to lighten her mood. "Look at the reflection of the willows in the water. I'm going to bring the kids here one day when the war is over."

The road we take winds through the forest, so we decide to hitchhike, but passing cars are rare, and most of them belong to UNPROFOR. We don't trust them, so we let them pass. Finally, a small Fiat with license plates from Glina comes rumbling along. It skids to a halt, the door opens, and a giraffe-like man emerges from the tiny car. *Get in!* he says. Dara and I hop in and we somehow managed to squeeze into the cramped back seat. The dashboard is falling apart and wires are dangling over the driver's knees. But we're overjoyed because he can get us right to the hospital even before the ambulance is supposed to leave to pick us up.

I've been feeling guilty about using up the hospital's precious gasoline, so hitchhiking did the trick.

He barely managed to get the Fiat started again, but he did drive us all the way back to the hospital, where we thanked him profusely. The ambulance driver was surprised:

— What happened? Weren't you supposed to get your hair done?

Souls in Distress

As Yugoslavia disintegrated, the JNA disintegrated along with it. A meandering fault line separated the inhabitants in time and space — entire worlds disappeared. Many people became stateless because one country was abolished but no new country had yet been established to replace it. Personal history is being erased. Parents are leaving their children; children their parents. Husbands are leaving their wives; wives their husbands. And friendships are ending. People are clinging to settled-upon solutions like leeches. In order to cope, one has to escape this terrifying whirlwind of personal wishes, memories, and fixed opinions. Many people suffer physical harm, others suffer disorientation and misery. We're all waiting for the confused situation to sort itself out.

History is repeating itself. It takes a hundred years to establish a family, but the single stroke of a pen at a negotiating table is all it takes to destroy it. Does the UN actually believe that sanctions are going to help people?

Dušan is a JNA soldier, a sniper. We got acquainted at one of the social events held at the hospital. He was born in a village that now, after the partition, belongs to Croatia. He and his young family don't live there anymore, but his elderly parents decided to stay — even die, if necessary — on their native land. Dušan's wife is Croatian. They have a son. At the beginning of the war, her parents moved to Belgrade from Zagreb. No one bothered them there. Meanwhile, Croats were harassing and killing Serbs in Zagreb. This is terribly hard on Dušan, who's a Serb. He has no contact with his parents. He fears for their safety. So as soon as he safely relocated his wife and family to Belgrade, he rejoined his Special Forces unit in Krajina, where he took part in a number of successful raids.

He shows up at our party with friends from JNA headquarters. He joins our efforts to break up the monotony and dispel our persistent sense of fear. He picks up an accordion and, at first, plays and sings timidly. Then he spreads the bellows and suddenly plaintive sounds fill the room. One song follows after another, and we huddle together, embracing each other. Dušan unites us by conjuring a clear expression of intangible suffering.

He's exhausted on top of being half drunk, so we relieve him of his accordion and I take him to a room where he can sleep it off. He goes silently, leaning on me all the way to the room. A colleague helps him take off his shoes and get him into bed.

"I don't want to fall asleep," he says. "I'm afraid to go to sleep! Whenever I close my eyes, I see my home, my parents at the doorstep...."

Suddenly, he's sober. He starts telling his story.

"My mother and father are looking at me reproachfully, and they're saying: *You've abandoned us, Dušan. This is your house. This is where your childhood is. This is where you learned to walk, son. This is where you uttered your first words....*"

Dušan covers his face with his hands and begins weeping.

"Believe me! I wanted to bring them there — take them to Belgrade," he continues. "But they didn't want to be refugees in their old age. They swore that they would rather die in their own home. I'm afraid they might die a violent death. Their neighbors are good people, but others, whose intentions may not be good, can show up at any time and then everything would be over in a few seconds. The Croats put me on a list of war criminals, so that makes matters even worse for my mother and father."

"I understand how hard this is for you, but I admire your parents," I say spontaneously. "They're real people."

"They're wonderful people," he replies. "They're proud, and their pride is killing me. How could I leave them like that? It's winter, and they're old. They don't have any money, and they can't afford to buy fuel. I'm worried about them and it's driving me crazy. I keep seeing them looking chilblained, hungry, or maybe murdered. I took my wife's Croatian parents with me, but I left my own parents behind!"

"You didn't leave them behind. They chose to stay," I say. "They have the right to make their own decision, and to choose their life or death. You need to get some sleep. You'll look at things differently tomorrow."

"You don't understand!" he says, still agitated. "I can't calm down until my village becomes part of Krajina again. It's only ten kilometers from here. Only ten kilometers separate me from my mother and father, from my past. Damn this war!" he cries, his face writhing with pain.

"Whenever I go into action, I imagine I'm liberating my village. I asked my commander a hundred times to take those ten kilometers. He said it was impossible. There was an agreement. I can't accept that. I'm going to fight my own war! Against all of them on both sides!"

A spasm wracks Dušan's face, then he falls asleep. Who annihilated his forest, his stream, his childhood?

We haven't seen or heard from him since. People said he had been discharged for insubordination.

After I returned to Belgrade, my friends told me that Dušan had been killed. He took his sniper rifle and went off to fight his own private war. He was killed by a Croatian sniper almost in front of the house where he was born. And that was where he died.

Why?

Yugoslavia 1945

The Kingdom of Serbs, Croats and Slovenes was proclaimed in 1918 as a bulwark against German expansionism. The post-WWII Yugoslav state was composed of six republics and two autonomous regions (Vojvodina and Kosovo).

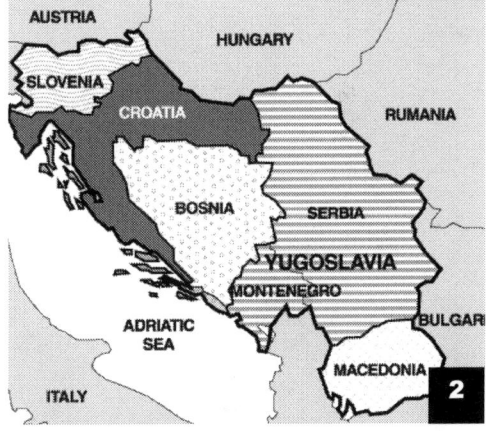

Yugoslavia 1991

Germany breaks up Yugoslavia as it did during WWII. Serbia was weakened by embargos and secessions. Croatia becomes an independent country as it was briefly during WWII when it was allied with Nazi Germany. Kosovo will later be detached from Serbia as it was during WWII.

The Republika Srpska Krajina
(areas in black)

In response to Croatia's illegally obtained independence, Serbs living in Croatia proclaimed the independence of the Republika Srpska Krajina, which was not granted international recognition. The RSK government fought for unification with the Republika Srpska in Bosnia and Serbia.

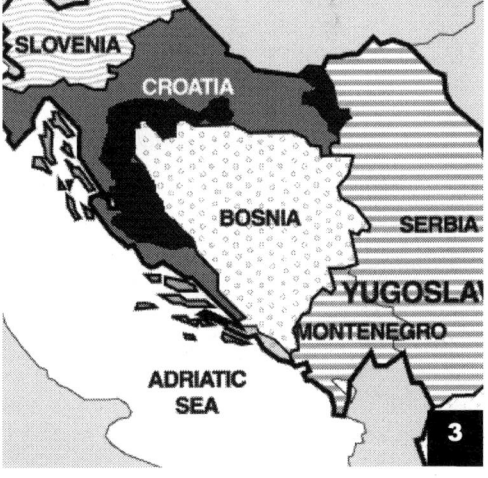

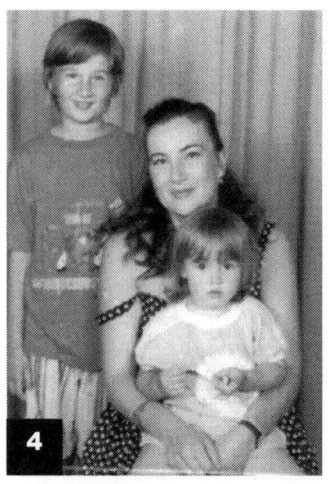

Dr. Mitic with her daughters on the eve of the war

I'm awakened by howling dogs. Their baying vacillates, at one moment near, at another far. I think about my children. This damned war, I think. I simply had to come. It's my duty as a physician, but I'm still upset about having left my children. I try to bring my mind back to my reality, where my struggle for peace must begin. (p. 99)

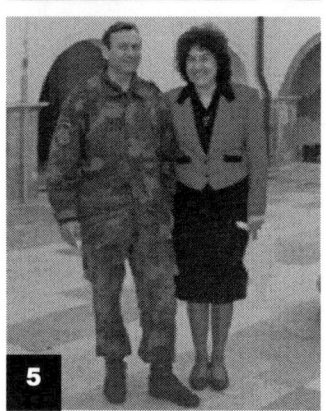

Dr. Mitic with Commander Vrcelj

Colonel Vrcelj spent most of his adult life as a soldier in Slovenia. He left behind everything he had there. Long before the war, he sensed trouble brewing, so he warned the JNA leadership that something strange was going on in Slovenia.... But the leadership ignored his warnings. Now we're all being punished for their blindness. (p. 129)

The Smederevo Fortress

The wind caressed my face. I could hear the voices of those who built this fortress with the last atom of their strength in order to protect Serbia from the Ottoman invasion. Their hands now rose out of the past and urged me forward. (p. 339)

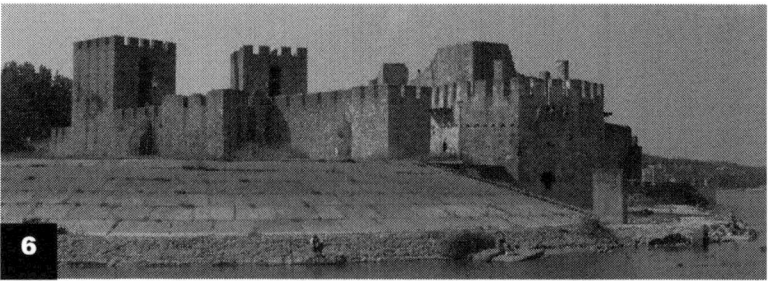

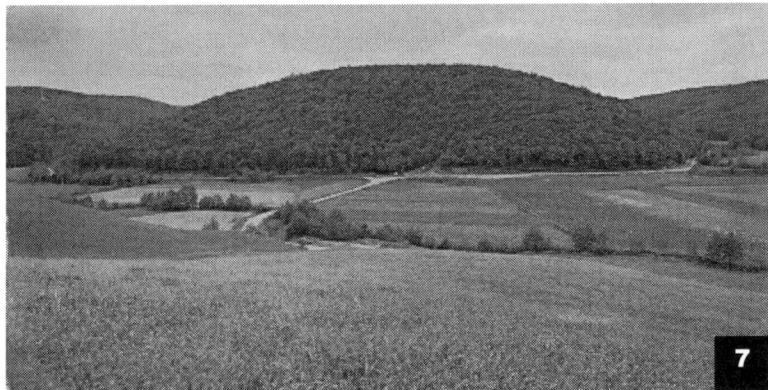

A panoramic view of Petrova Gora

The War Memorial

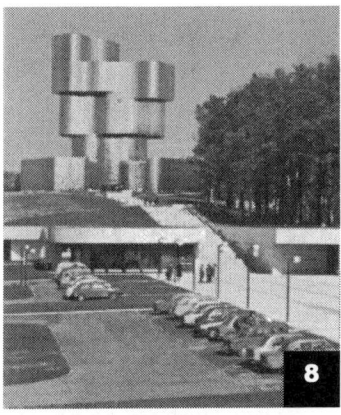

He withdrew to Petrova Gora with like-minded people. Dr. Dragojevic, a fellow surgeon who was also from Karlovac, joined him. The two of them and an otolaryngologist established the first war hospital in Petrova Gora. At an altitude of 500 meters, beside the war memorial erected in honor of the victims of Fascism during WWII, yet another war hospital was set up in wooden shacks. Memories of WWII are still palpable in this dense forest of chestnut, oak, and beech trees.

A village near Petrova Gora

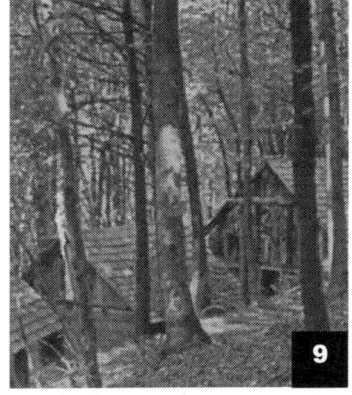

A steep and winding road leads to the hospital. It's difficult to reach after a snowfall. These are nineteenth-century conditions: no electricity, no reliable water supply, and no adequate heating. The physicians still manage to function somehow. Wounded soldiers keep arriving along with civilians whose illnesses require medical treatment. We save lives. (p. 108)

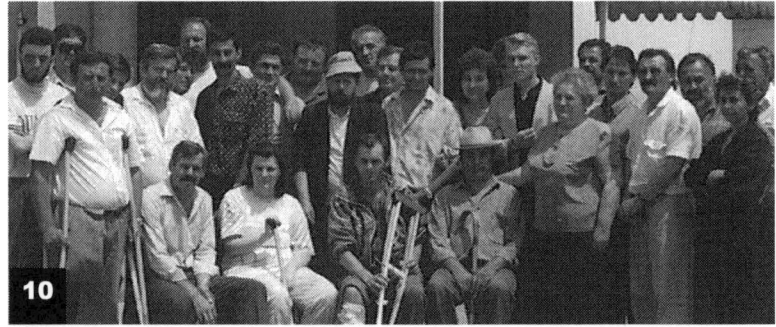

Members of the Invalid War Veterans Assoc. in Smederevo
By arrangement with the hospital director, we established a shelter for psychologically traumatized and mentally-handicapped veterans who had returned from the battlefield. Our psychologist took on a huge burden. All of these men remain traumatized. Two tried to kill themselves with explosives; later, six others tried to hang themselves. (p. 79)

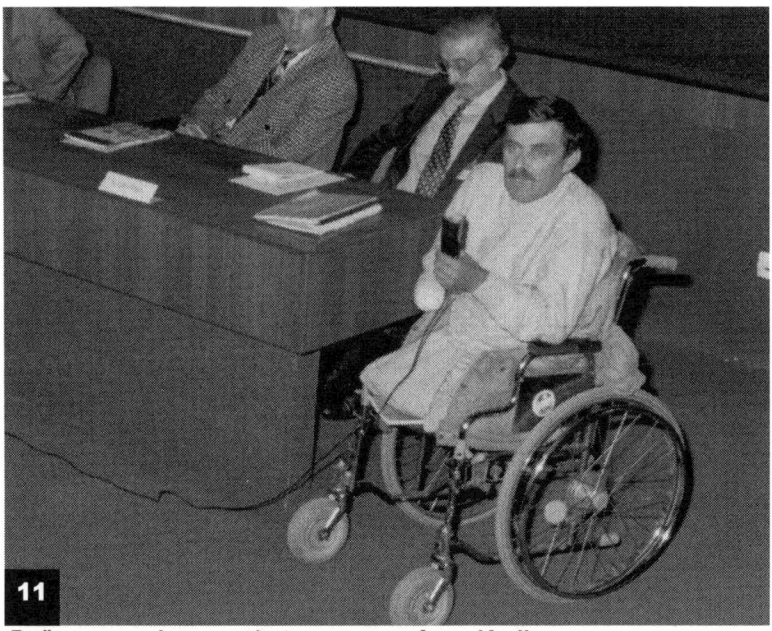

Dušan, a sculptor and stonemason from Krajina.
A bomb had blown his legs off, along with an arm and an eye. He's crippled for life but he remains of sound mind and he has a phenomenal will to live. He continues to paint. On the one hand, he's expending creative energy, which rescues him from boredom; but on the other hand, it's a constant reminder of all the things he can no longer do.
(p. 265)

Jihad against Serbs

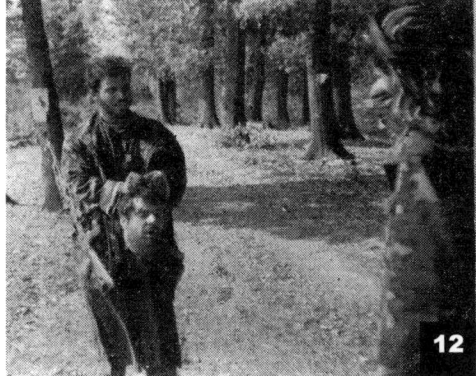

Halil Abaz Aziz, a mujahideen figher from Saudi Arabia, holding the decapitated head of a Serbian soldier. The unprocessed film containing these photos was found on the person of Aziz, who was himself killed in a firefight in August 1992.

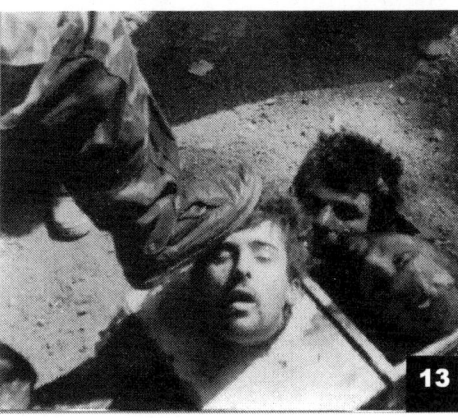

Aziz plants his foot triumphantly on the heads of slain Serbs.

A Serbian priest beside the ruins of his church in Petrinje.
Serbia is being attacked from all directions. Television screens unleash terrifying images of fire, devastation, charred human remains, and the demolished homes of ordinary people who, if they survive, now have nowhere to go. (p. 290)

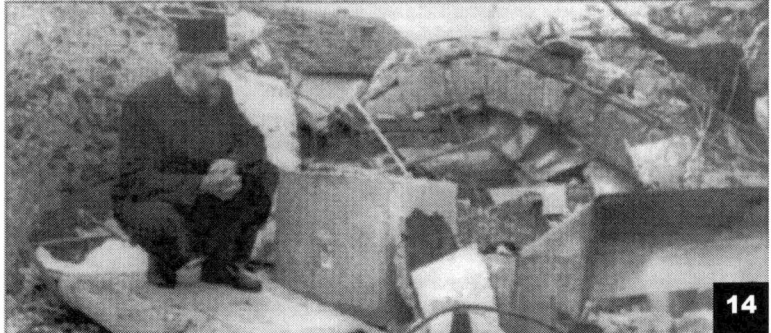

The charred remains of Milomir Prodanovic, from Podravanje near Milici in Bosnia

The smoke from this evil fire was rising into the sky. There was a man impaled on the spit. His abdomen had been ripped open. It was Murad's incision and all his entrails were hanging out, and some had fallen into the ashes. Blood was still oozing, and the poor man was still alive. His eyes were swollen and his skin, a red-black color, was cracked all over.

He whispered: "If you're Serbs… if you've got a heart … kill me!" (p. 90)

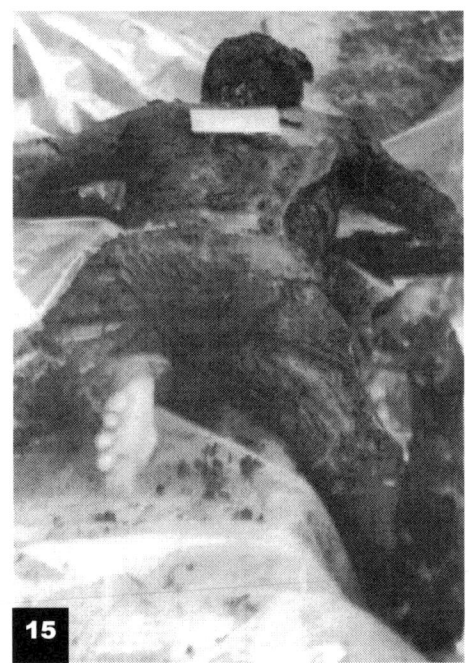

Serbian RSK soldiers from Knin leaving for battle
The likelihood of bombardment had been plaguing us for days beforehand. Knin is situated in a valley. There is no way out except by the main roads. Shellfire and explosions from the surrounding areas reverberate throughout the entire valley. (p. 42)

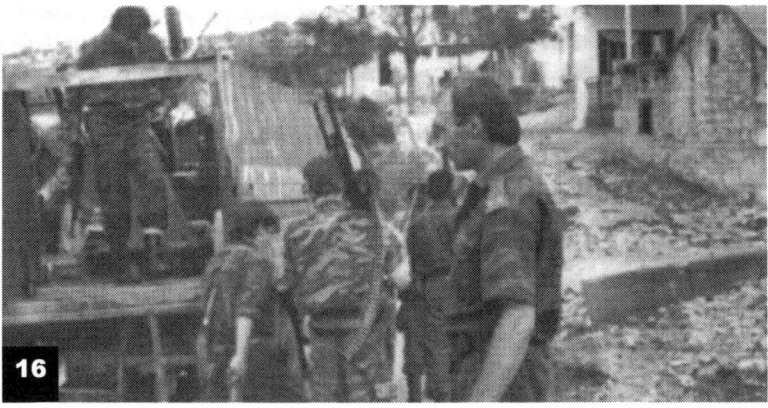

Refugees from Knin

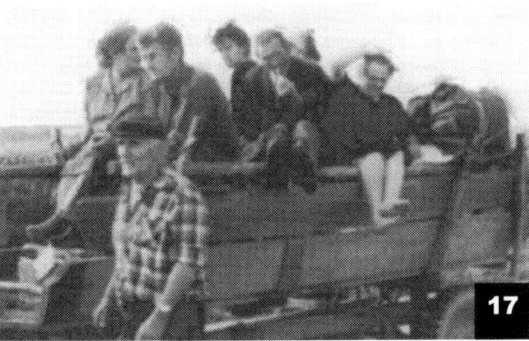

The refugees' miserable belongings are piled on a somber procession of tractors: bundles of clothing, footwear, and white pressure cookers are easily be distinguished. The women have wrinkled faces that seem to have grown old overnight; they have dull, absent expressions, and they are staring blankly into the distance because they have left their souls behind in the homes they abandoned. They are traveling into the unknown, leaving the places where they were born, where they married, where they gave birth to their children. They wouldn't have had time to feed or water their livestock; their houses have been left open. Their homes don't belong to them anymore. Someone turned a leaf in the Doomsday Book, which resulted in their lives being hurled into a dark abyss. Are their Croatian neighbors going to take care of those homes until the war is over? The column of people stretches into a long undulating line over the countryside.(p. 30)

Refugees from Republika Srpska Krajina arrive in Serbia

From that moment on, it was each man for himself. People coped as well as they could in conditions of utter chaos. Throughout Bosnia, which had its own problems, columns of refugees were wandering down roads that led to salvation in Banja Luka. One group arrived at a border crossing with Serbia in a jalopy that had neither a windshield nor a rear window. The car was falling apart as they were driving it. They were pale with shock and covered with blood and dust. After crossing the border into Serbia, each went his own way. At first, they were only interested in saving their own lives. Now, as I'm listening to them, I'm not even sure whether their own lives were still important to them.

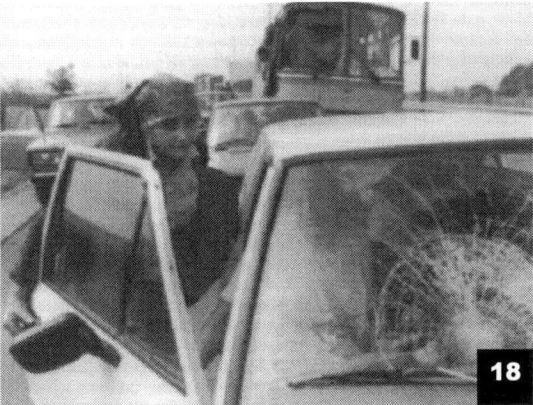

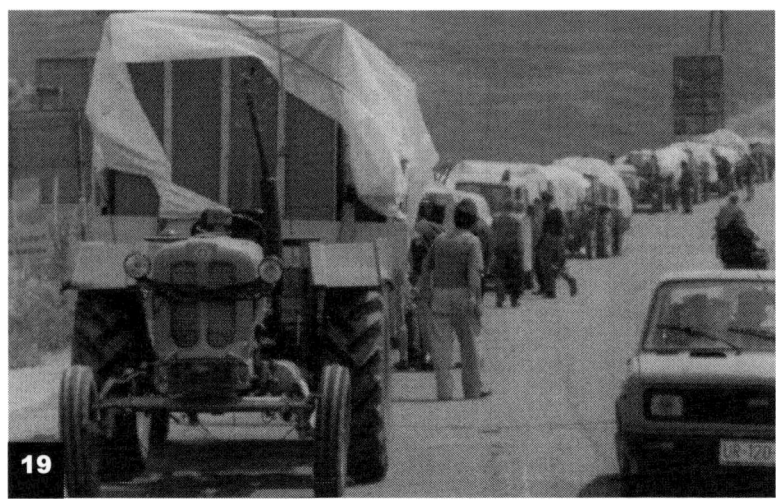

Serbian refugees fleeing Kosovo during the 1999 bombardment
The next day, thirty of us set out for Kosovo in two cars and a minibus while the inhabitants of Kosovo are leaving. We're going against an endless line of poor people who are driving tractors loaded with luggage and household possessions. I saw similar columns of refugees back in Krajina in 1991, and again in 1995 when two hundred thousand of the last Serbs in Croatia drove, ran, and walked to Serbia. Now a similar column of refugees is fleeing Kosovo. It's heartbreaking to see the disheveled and disorganized members of paramilitary forces who joined this column. But we're going to Kosovo. (p. 329)

April 3, 1999, about 7:50 p.m.
The destroyed Liberty Bridge, Novi Sad -- Sremska Kamenica. The NATO agressors fired three missiles that hit the Liberty Bridge. One missile strick the middle, while the others demolished the part of the bridge leading to the bank on Srem. Five persons were severely wounded, and three others were wounded.

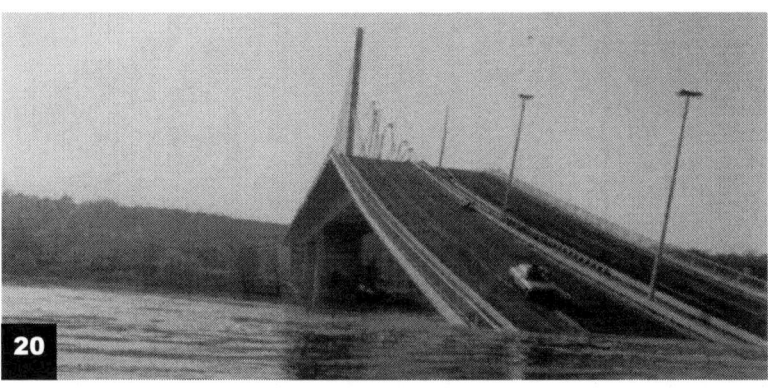

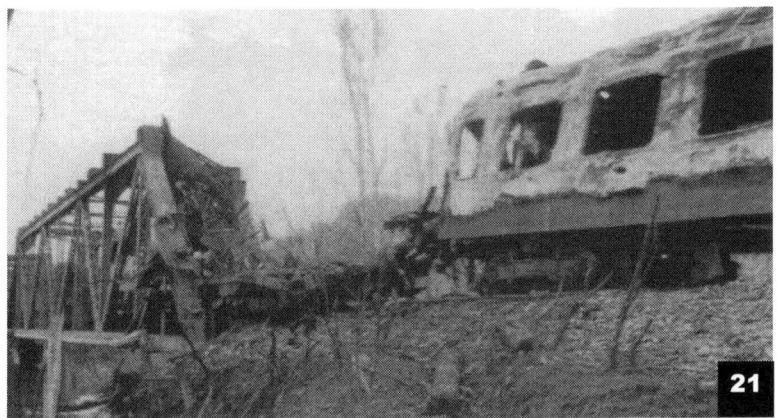

April 12, 1999, 11:40 a.m.
NATO warplanes destroyed the 'Sarajevo' Railway Bridge and passanger train No. 393 near the town of Grdelica. This attack targeted civilians: nine passengers were killed and sixteen injurerd. The missiles also destroyed the coaxial telephone cable, which cut off telephone communications with southern Serbian, Macedonia, and Greece.

April 23, 1999, 2:20 a.m.
NATO warplanes targeted the Radio-Television Serbia (RTS) building in downtown Belgrade. Six bodies were pulled out of the wreckage, another seventeen were listed as missing. Sixteen other persons received medical assistance for minor injuries.

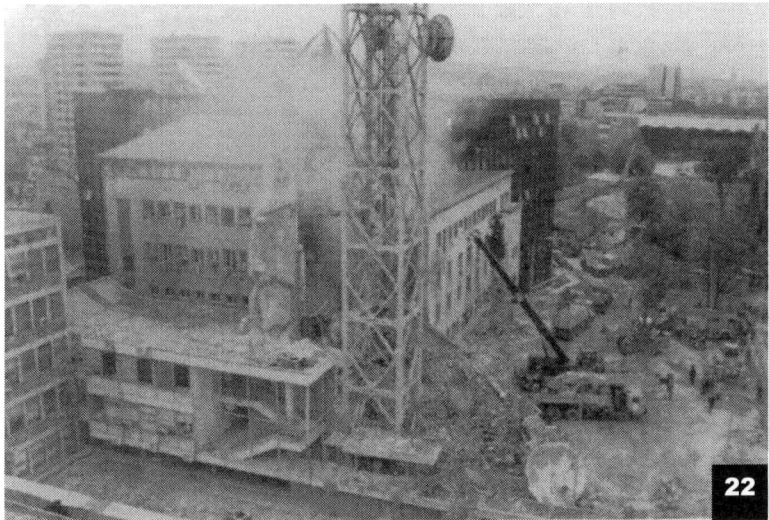

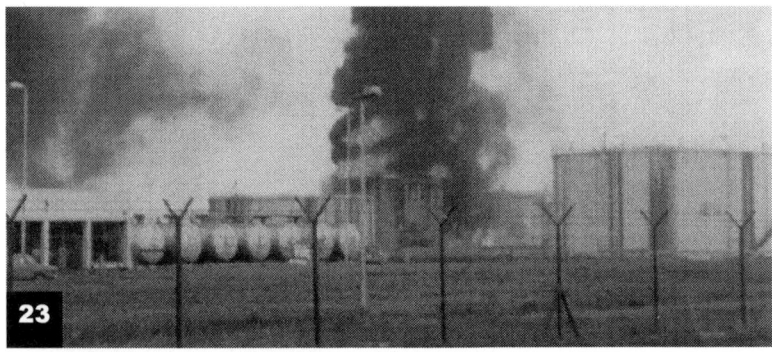

Smederevo, April 9, 1999
Six missiles hit NIS Jugopetrol. Five missiles struck tanks with oil and oil by-products (kerosene, petrol).
As I leave my building, I'm dazzled by powerful light emanating from the Kovin Bridge, where smoke and flames are belching into the dark sky. The conflagration is lighting up the whole town. A missile hit the Jugopetrol Oil Reserves refinery, which burst into flames. I can't tell if there are any casualties. I also wonder why I didn't hear the explosion. I must have been dead asleep. (p. 288)

Nis, May 7, 1999
Between 11:30 a.m. and 11:40 a.m., NATO aircraft dropped two containers of cluster bombs on Nis. One fell in front of the Pathology Clinic in the south-eastern part of town; the other fell in the city center close to the University of Nis Rectorate. These bomblets killed thirteen persons. Below is the body of Ljiljana Spasic (1973), seven-months pregnant, who was killed on the corner of Jelena Dimitrijevic and Sumatovacka Streets.

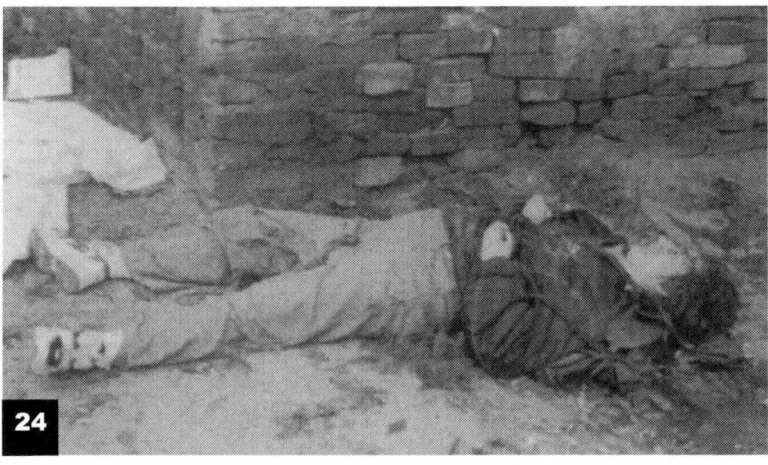

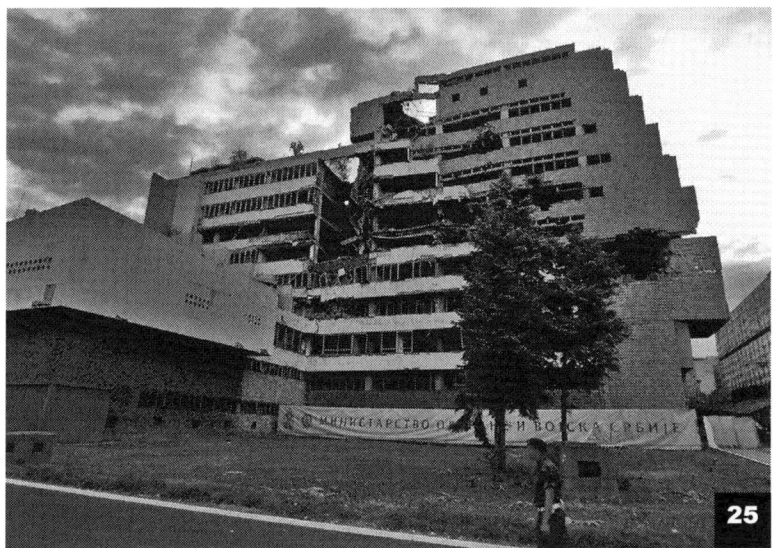

General Staff of the Yugoslav Army in Belgrade, April 29-30

A black mushroom cloud rises from the direction of Army Headquarters. Whorls of smoke rise from the lower floors as sharp, yellow flames lick the sides of the building. O, my God, is this an atomic bomb?! The scene resembles Hiroshima. I can't believe it. I'm paralyzed by shock, but another more distressing thought flashes through my mind. I know Marko is near the Army Headquarters. (p. 312)

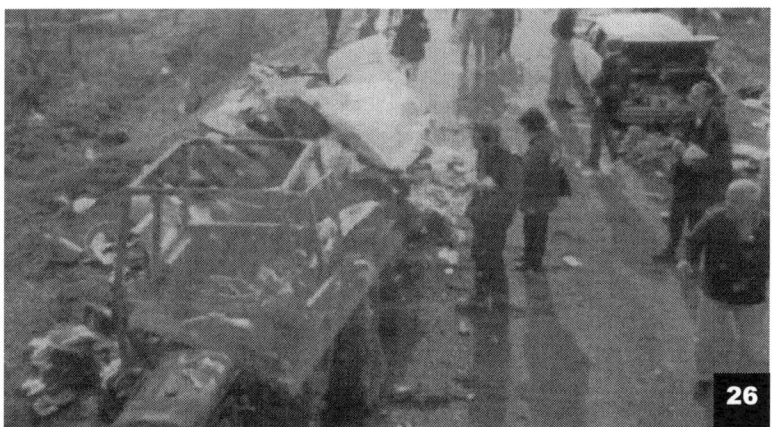

April 14, 1999

Today NATO bombed a column of Albanian refugees. About a hundred old men, women, and children were killed. It was dreadful! .... NATO deliberately bombed these poor people. There's no other explanation. Did they think that the tractors belonged to Serbs...? (p. 297)

Photo Credits

1 Collon, Michel. *Liar's Poker: The Great Powers, Yugoslavia, and the Wars of the Future*. New York: IAC, 2002.

2 Ibid.

3 Ibid., note that map was modified to show territory of RSK.

4 Author's personal collection

5 Ibid.

6 Government of Serbia Tourist Agency

7 Ivan Grgić

8 Photographer unknown

9 Photographer unknown

10 Author's personal collection

11 Ibid.

12 From "Genocide against the Serbs," a photography exhibition curated by Bojana Isaković in 1992

13 Ibid.

14 Seklulić, Milisav. *Knin je pao u Beograd*. Bad Vilbel: Nidda Verlag GmbH, 2000.

15 Jovanović, Drago et al. *The Eradication of the Serbs in Bosnia and Herzegovina 1992–1993*. Beograd: IP RAD, 1995.

16 *Knin je pao u Beograd, op. cit.*

17 Ibid.

18 Ibid.

19 Andjelković, Zoran et al. *Days of Terror (in the Presence of the International Forces)*. Belgrade: Center for Peace and Tolerande, 2000.

20 Federal Ministry of Foreign Affairs. *NATO Crimes in Yugoslavia: Documentary Evidence 24 March – 24 April 1999*. Belgrade: Federal Republic of Yugoslavia, 1999.

21 Ibid.

22 Ibid.

23 Ibid.

24 Ibid.

25 Photographer unknown

26 *NATO Crimes in Yugoslavia: Documentary Evidence 24 March – 24 April 1999, op. cit.*

PART THREE

19. I Leave One War for Another

In June 1993, about six months after I had begun working in Glina, I finally returned to Serbia.

A hundred people came to my farewell party. Dr. Dario delivered a touching speech. When it was my turn to speak, tears were streaming from my eyes. All I could say was: "I'll come back. I love you!"

I'm never going to forget the doctors and the nurses I worked with. I'll always think of them with pride as well as with sadness.

The OR called in the middle of the party. A group of soldiers had returned safely from Dalmatia. They were celebrating and firing gunshots in the air when one of them was accidentally shot by friendly fire. The operation lasted the whole night. The nurses were waiting for me in the half-light of dawn to say good-bye. I was exhausted. They were holding some packages they had wrapped for me: keepsakes. We embraced each other quietly for a long time.

Commander Marko Vrcelj, who was also traveling with his son Vladamir to Belgrade, brought me back to reality. The minibus, a military vehicle, was ready to leave.

"Come on, Doctor! We've got a long drive ahead."

I boarded with the other passengers and sat next to Colonel Vrcelj. I waved good-bye again. Then I turned around and buried my head in Marko's chest and sobbed. He caressed me gently.

"Easy does it," he whispered, consoling me.

I slept for more than half the trip. Luckily, our long drive transpired without incident despite the constant threat of an attack. With 800 km of road behind us, I awoke just as we were entering Belgrade.

I have not seen my children for six months. I fret about how they are going to react to my returning home. Are they going to hold a grudge against me for having been absent so long? I had initially gone only for a month, but ended up staying all winter and well into the spring. I also promise to take Marko's son Vladimir to live with us until his situation settled down. Vladimir had nowhere to go because Marko's current wife is not Vladimir's mother. She doesn't want to take any responsibility for the boy.

I'm also afraid of what condition my apartment is going to be in. Has anyone been taking care of it? Where is Miroslav? Is he with this new lady friend? I'm annoyed by the legal matters that are awaiting me. One more divorce — one more personal failure.

I felt safe as I was sleeping on Marko's shoulder. Now, upon entering Belgrade, I'm fully awake and I realize we have to part ways again. Even in Krajina, I didn't get to see him every day, but here we're facing new obstacles. Marko's wife will be waiting for him in Belgrade. I, of course, have my own problems.

Marko hugs me gently; my heartbeat picks up.

"After you drop off all the passengers," he says to the driver, "let's give the Doctor a lift back to Smederevo. She deserves that much. She saved quite a few lives. We should show our appreciation."

How am I going to part with Marko? Yet I yearn for my children. I desperately want to take a hot bath and go to sleep without the sounds of distant artillery fire. That's all behind me now, but I've left one war only to step right into another. When we reach my building in Smederevo, Marko carries my suitcases up the stairs.

Scrawled across the door of my apartment is a huge cross and the year "1994" written beneath it. That's another death threat Miroslav has received. I try my keys but they don't work. After several attempts, it becomes clear the locks have been changed. I'm too embarrassed to even look at Marko.

"You should have expected that," he says matter-of-factly. "What are you going to do now?"

"My neighbors agreed to wait for me," I say, feeling the tears welling up in my eyes. "I should check with them."

Marko caresses my cheek and reassures me. Then I see my neighbors coming down the hall. Nada, who is secretary to the president of the municipal government, arrives with her husband, Slobodan. They're joined by another couple, Tanja and Slavko. They ask me:

"Where have you been?"

"We were about to lose hope!"

"We began thinking that they weren't going to let you leave!"

I introduce Marko to them and they welcome him warmly as a man who has both served in and survived battlefields. Nada and Slobodan take my suitcase, and they tell me that I'll be spending the night with them.

Awaiting us is a table set with a variety of dishes. I haven't seen so much food in a long time. It smells wonderful, but I'm not really hungry. I can't bring myself to ask about my apartment, so I downplay my concerns. They're happy I'm alive, and I'm touched by their genuine concern. They aren't going to allow Marko to leave without joining us for lunch, so he fetches Vladimir as well as the driver. Soon after that, my daughters appear at the door. They've been at their nanny's home. I shed tears of joy and I embraced them a long while.

It's a festive occasion. Marko loves company and he tells amusing stories. We laugh a great deal. But reality is never far from my conscious mind: I'm alone again. What am I going to do with my children? How am I going to take care of Vladimir? We have no place to live. The locked door of my apartment isn't going to reveal any more of the story.

It was only after Marko returned Belgrade that I found out what had happened during my absence. Miroslav had moved from our apartment and had gone to live with the woman I read about in the papers. She's a pharmacist in our hospital. I know her. Other things had been happening behind the scenes. It was so complicated that I had no idea what was going to happen next.

I just wanted to get my life back with my children as soon as possible. But it wasn't easy. I had to go to court on numerous occasions just to get a permit to enter my apartment.

The presiding judge, who had once been a neighbor of mine, completely ignored me. As far as he was concerned, I had no rights to the apartment nor did I have any legal protection because I had voluntarily left my apartment to go to the front lines. In his opinion, my husband had the legal right to keep the apartment should we divorce. I didn't know how to reach Miroslav to resolve the matter. I was frightened by these procedures, frightened by the menacing cross on our door, and frightened by the convoluted information I was getting about Miroslav. He promised to protect me and the children; he promised that our destiny would not be his, but I knew I had to stay away from him in order to keep myself and my children safe.

Just a couple of days later, my friends from the police department helped me enter the apartment so I could get my checkbook and some personal belongings.

During the first week, I stayed with Nada and Slobodan. I went back to work at the hospital in Smederevo. I didn't have anything to wear because I had given away all my usable clothing in Krajina. I knew it was going to be easier for me to buy new clothes than it would be for them. My neighbors lent me some clothes, so I had at least something to wear when I had to go to work, to court, and to the police station.

A judge finally ruled that I could enter my apartment. Miroslav had begun legal action against me while I was still in Krajina. The divorce papers had already been filed in court. Despite that, he did come to the apartment one night and he begged me to pack my bags and take the children and go to my uncle in Canada.

"Please, understand," he begs. "This is going to cost me plenty. The only way to avoid getting killed is to escape. You have to get away, too. The Serbian MUP (*i.e.*, Ministry of Internal Affairs, the security services) will track you down and execute you if they identify you as having been involved with me. I'm a first-hand witness to financial improprieties being committed by people in power. In other words, I'm an obstacle that has to be eliminated."

Miroslav looks desperate. He has gone pale with fear. It's hard for me to see him like this. I hold his hands. They're warm and sweaty. I hold him tight, so he can feel my sadness. I look deep into his beautiful green eyes. I can't think about going away. No one in Canada has invited us to come. My head and my heart are confused.

He begins crying too. We end up lying on the floor of the apartment, crying together. We hold hands so tightly that it begins to hurt. Luckily, the children aren't at home. They love Miroslav and they don't understand his prolonged absence.

I remember speaking to them about it. *Mom, why doesn't Cile love you anymore?* asked my youngest daughter. *You're more beautiful than his new wife. I'll tell him that he just can't leave us like that.*

Ljuba, honey! I replied, trying to explain in terms that she could understand. *Mom left Cile alone by himself for a long time. It's only natural. These things happen!*

But Mom, somebody had to help save all those children in Krajina and all those other people. I have to explain this to Cile, she kept saying.

I'm looking at Miroslav's face again.

"Look after the children," he begs me. "You have to protect them. There's no way out for me, even if I resign."

Then Miroslav gets up and leaves. I never saw him privately again. The only other time I saw him again was in court at the divorce hearing. Miroslav had supposedly asked me during a telephone conversation while I was in Krajina to agree to start divorce proceedings. He allegedly implored me to return to Serbia. He had recorded the conversation, but I couldn't remember having had any such conversation at all. Who had he been talking to? What did this mean? Our divorce was sensationalized, which made it easier for me to distance myself emotionally. It was a relief when it was all over.

* * * *

Now it's March 1994. March 8, 1990 is the anniversary of our first date. I was the physician who had been assigned to treat his younger brother during abdominal surgery. Miroslav was always there during his brother's recovery. He invited me to lunch so he could thank me for my kindness and my efforts on behalf of his brother. I helped out his entire family by giving them free medical advice. He sent me flowers for the first time on March 8. He had stopped his car on a whim in front of a flower shop in Belgrade. He returned with a large red flamingo. He told me it was called an anthurium. We used to observe this anniversary by dining out in a restaurant. Now, on March 8, 1994, I feel the sudden stab of heartfelt pain because I'm not going to see him.

* * * *

I went for a walk and saw his car, which was, in fact, our car because we hadn't yet divided our property. It was parked in front of the apartment building where his mother was living, but he wasn't there. No one had seen him for several days. When the police came to see me at the hospital on March 12, two days later, I knew that they had found him.

They took me to his office, which was right across the street from the courthouse and the police station, where Miroslav had begun his career as an attorney. This was where his body was found lying on the floor. He was wearing his raincoat, the one he usually wore over his suit. He always looked as if he had just come in or was about to go out. His big green eyes were vacant;

his lips half-open, as if he wanted to say something. I felt tears coming on. I knelt beside his body and embraced him. His head wobbled left, then right. His neck had been broken. The whites of his eyes still shone; his retina still carried an image of laughter and high-jinx. I recalled him pleading with me to flee the country, and I recalled his words about escape being the only way to avoid being killed. I listened calmly, albeit with a growing sense of rigidity, to the policeman as he explained that he had been found hanged in the bathroom. The rope around his neck had three tight bowline knots. The killers must have broken into his office. I looked at his neck but saw no telltale furrow that a hanged man always has. His eyeballs and tongue were in place. He had definitely not been hanged. Miroslav had weak, feminine hands. He couldn't have tied a bowline knot. He was actually ashamed of it because he did own a boat, which he liked to brag about. He just couldn't have tied the three strong bowline knots that allegedly ended his life.

The coroner, who came to write up the official death certificate, doubted that it was suicide, even though the police had ordered him to write *Suicide* as the cause of death on the death certificate. He resisted:

"But I can't lie!" he pleaded.

I glared at him and said:

"Can you bring him back to life? No, you can't! Can lose your life? Yes, you can! I'm afraid for myself as well as for my children, and I'm afraid for your life, too. This is no joke. Miroslav had been warned a long time ago that this was coming."

I had been told before his death to buy a coffin. Scrawled on our door was a cross along with the year 1994. It was March 1994, and he was dead.

We buried Miroslav the next day. There was no autopsy, no medical examination, no nothing. We placed his body in the coffin right in his office. We took him to the chapel at the cemetery.

I spent several hours there holding vigil over his body. Three thousand people attended his funeral. Our car, which had been parked on the street right in front of the police station, was stolen during the funeral. No one will ever know what was hidden inside the car.

After the funeral, silence set in. People were scared. Soon afterward, two more people were killed in a similar fashion in Smederevo, as well as others all over Serbia. The well-known journalist Dada Vujašinović was killed. The daughter of General Mladić, the Commander of Army of the Republika Srpska, allegedly committed suicide. I don't believe any of these stories. Suicide is an unimaginative way of dealing with dissent.

Miroslav — A.K.A. Cile

Miroslav came into my life when I was alone with two small children in a new city. I was a divorced single mother, a doctor, and I had demanding hours at the hospital. I didn't even have my own apartment. I was living in a rented apartment in Smederevo. I was also the first on the list of hospital staff eligible for an apartment. For personal reasons, the hospital director changed my ranking, so I dropped to the number two spot. This also meant that we had to leave the apartment where we were living.

It was February 1990. The streets were icy, so it was dreadfully slippery and terribly cold. Frosty isolation permeated every aspect of my life. I didn't have any help, and I didn't know where to go with two small children on the salary I earned as a resident physician, which was insufficient. As these ominous clouds were gathering, Miroslav appeared and came to the rescue. He was part of the establishment, so people wielding power in positions of authority lent him support. Above all, he was sympathetic to me as well as to my dilemma. He wanted to help. I didn't have a choice but to accept.

My relationship with my family had been strained recently because I divorced a husband with whom I had irreconcilable differences. My family considered the institution of marriage to be sacred. The wife had to endure anything and everything, even physical abuse. I would not tolerate violence, so divorce was inevitable. Keeping my integrity was of the utmost importance, but I paid dearly for it. I was alone and desperate when Miroslav extended the hand of friendship. I knew I could rely on him. He was intelligent. He helped me come back down to earth. And he taught me more about life and people than I had known up until then. Books had always been my best friends and I was always an outstanding student, but I was inept in my personal affairs. My judgment of character, especially of men, was always mistaken. My head was in the clouds!

Miroslav was indispensable because he taught me what my family hadn't. Miroslav helped heal my wounds and he taught me survival strategies. He loved life. I'll always remember the things he said. I'll also remember his predictions — more precisely, his accurate analyses of various emerging events. They were right on the money because the test of time has proven them true.

On the one hand, Miroslav was unusually intelligent; on the other hand, he was sensitive and vulnerable, which often made him emotionally unpredictable and difficult. His passionate temperament led him to express things in strong emotional terms. Miroslav lived every day as if it were his last. He enjoyed every moment of his life and he taught me and my children to enjoy the simple things. That was not my strong suit. I was defined by an intense work life. I was a person who only worked and then worked some more. He taught me how to relax.

The children loved him. We traveled across Serbia together, so we saw our country from different perspectives. Miroslav loved everything. He loved his car as if it were a woman. He loved to eat, he loved to drink, he loved to dance, and he loved to sing. He used to come home, toss his briefcase aside, and immediately start dancing. Half of his genes came from his Chilean mother, which made him want to get up and dance. I learned how to drop whatever I was doing and start dancing with him. The children also danced with us, and soon we were all laughing. Every day was a joy.

When we were traveling through Zlatibor, a mountain range in western Serbia, he would let go of the steering wheel and spread his arms wide.

"Look at this natural beauty," he'd say. "Nowhere else in the world can you find anything like it! But evil people want to destroy it. Look! This is Serbia. This is the true Serbia: fertile land, sloping mountains, lush forests. Remember, this is the real Serbia!"

Miroslav often recounted his adventures in the courtroom. Before he became the Director of the Public Revenue Office, he had served as a judge and as a defense attorney. He defended engineers from the steel mills after equipment breakdowns. I would pretend that I had come before a judge, and then he demonstrated the whole process. It was a riveting experience. He took pride in winning cases against the state. He was always outspoken. He wasn't at all circumspect in his public remarks. He spoke against Draža Marković, who was the President of the League of Communists of Serbia at the time. He said that he was a drunken fool. He really was but no one dared to say it publicly. A person could lose his life for saying something like that. But someone did remember the remark, and Miroslav soon had the secret police knocking on his door. Miroslav said he had only been kidding, yet this incident dogged him as it was to dog me, too, from the moment he came into my life. Living with him meant sitting on a powder keg with a short fuse. If he didn't light the fuse himself, there was always someone around who would have been more than happy to light it for him.

Now I was no longer in the street as I had been when we first met. That was exactly what he had told me at the beginning of our relationship:

"Now you have nothing. But if we ever get divorced, remember that you'll get half of the apartment. And please remember that I've been in love with you for five years! That's why I'm helping you."

And there was something else — Cile loved justice.

"If you had been arm candy for some big shot, you would've gotten an apartment a long time ago," he said. "No one appreciates professionalism in this country, but I hold it in high regard."

Now they couldn't throw me out of the apartment. I have Cile to thank for this.

20. Telling Our Story

My attraction to the front lines resembled a drug addiction. I knew it wasn't good for me and that I had to avoid it, but I became so attached to it that I couldn't live without it. Abstinence hurts more than commitment. Thinking about Krajina and the events taking place across the Drina preoccupied me. The end of my relationship with Miroslav, as well as the subsequent tragedy, was dwarfed when compared to the heartache I felt about Krajina. The anguish was much greater than ordinary distress caused by problems in the world beyond our borders. I was living everyday life as if Krajina were a live wire dangling above my head. I drew strength from it to go on.

Throughout these upheavals, I was struggling to save lives. It just came down to the struggle for existence, which was, from my point of view, the only authentic and morally correct value in life. My life doesn't have a purpose: it's a struggle for survival. I was exhilarated and over-performed on the front lines. Wherever death forms a black background, life there etches its clear white lines in a foreground figure. This is the only pure, moral act: fighting for life.

I'm anguished by Krajina. I'm heartbroken by Serbia's indifference. It became clear to me that all the battles in Krajina had been abandoned or lost, and that its people have been left to the mercy of a terrifyingly ambiguous enemy.

It's difficult at work. My colleagues disapproved of my volunteer work in Krajina. They complained that they had to work longer hours to cover my absence while I was enjoying my new-found celebrity. This nonsense doesn't faze me. The pain I feel is stronger than their opinions.

In addition to my two children, Marko's son Vladimir arrived soon after I got my apartment back. He was not safe in Krajina, so I brought him here. Somehow, the four of us manage to live comfortably. Vladimir started working in a bakery as an apprentice, so that the baker, a friend of mine, could offer him a job later. My friends do help me a great deal. Without them, I wouldn't be able to survive with three children. Marko is still on the front lines, so we speak only occasionally on the phone, which is just enough to sustain my illusions.

The magazine *Duga* published extracts from my war diary, but the people I know are unsympathetic. Gossip takes on a life of its own, and a new story comes out with each passing day. There is absolutely no understanding of the suffering and misfortune that has befallen us. One journalist ridiculed my patriotism publicly. She said that patriotism suited me "just as well as a mini skirt suits someone with fat legs." She characterized me as a peasant woman who had just gotten her first high-heeled shoes and was now stumbling in them. Her vitriolic scorn didn't offend me.

This went on day in, day out. As time went on, I remained silent. Then, sanctions were imposed on Serbia. I couldn't heat the apartment. My pay was so miserable that I couldn't afford to buy a half liter of milk. Aunt Jelena, a dear friend of mine, was the only one who comforted me. There were two or three more friends who helped out. Everyone is hard up, but they managed to spare something for me. I managed to get along somehow. I wasn't poverty-stricken because I had enough food for the children. Over the summer, I prepared vegetable and fruit preserves to make winter stores. I was overwhelmed by sadness.

I snapped out of this despair with the help of an unusual journalist, Boris Katić. He came with a pediatrician named Boba Stajević who had come out in opposition to the party in power. Boris was the outgoing and self-assured host of *Politika*'s radio program *Strictly Confidential: These Are the Nineties*. With his cowboy boots and long blond hair, he looked as though he had just stepped off the set of a Hollywood Western. He peered straight into my eyes and asked me if I had written the text, excerpts from my war diary that Dr. Stajević had given him. These diary passages unexpectedly found their way to Boba's hands. I was annoyed.

"I didn't write that diary," I protested. "Life itself wrote it. I was just the witness. I wrote what I saw and experienced. I'm not a writer. I didn't invent any of those scenes."

I never had a chance to tell my story, so this turned out to be the catharsis I badly needed. I aired all my grief and pent up fury during the five-hour program. The audience received me with understanding, and many listeners told the producer that I had touched on sensitive matters that had long been suppressed. Readings from my diary passages were interspersed with songs from the former Yugoslavia that we all once loved. I was moved and encouraged. When the broadcast ended, Boris Katić and I went out for *burek*, a Turkish-style meat pastry. We walked through the dark streets eating the fresh burek with grease dripping from our fingers. I had released the pent up stress and anger I had been feeling for years. I found the act of telling my story to be powerfully healing.

The next week, Vanja Bulić, who was a journalist for the magazine *Duga* — as well as the producer of the television program *Black Pearls* — wanted to interview me for his show. I asked my colleagues, who had been in Krajina's hell with me, whether I should do the show. I didn't want to do anything they disapproved of.

"You have to, Sarah!" they said. "You have to! We don't have the gift of eloquence."

So, I told my story again. Vanja presented my report cards from school, awards for essay writing, distinctions I received in biology, and medals that I had won in competitive sports. He wanted to show that it wasn't just criminals who had gone to war, but "good guys" too. I was expecting the critics to tear me to shreds. But this time there were no arrogant critiques. Instead, my words awakened an unexpected flood of emotion in the audience. Strangers raised their voices to support and encourage me.

I was no longer alone.

21. Loving Sun and Stone

I had been in Krajina for months on end, but I was only able to leave the hospitals in which I had been working on a few isolated occasions. In 1991 and 1992, the situation in Knin was so dangerous that we were only able to leave the hospital — even if it meant just to take a walk — at our own risk. I didn't know anyone well enough to ask to join me in exploring the surrounding area, so those four years cast a long shadow over my life. I felt as though I was a thousand years old. I was more mature and experienced, and perhaps braver, but I was protected by a shield of indifference. Yet I longed to find out more about my mother's family because I knew Banija and Kordun better than I did Lika, the region where my mother was born.

My mother was raised in these high and daunting mountains above Knin. I didn't know where her family had originated, but I did know that she had come here as an infant. My mother's family had been forced to move many times. After World War II, her family moved to Slavonija during the so-called Eighth Offensive[18] when Tito's government forcibly resettled refugees. My grandmother used to tell us that they had been forced to move because they had been wealthy before the Communist government confiscated their property. Since they were hard-working and industrious, they acquired new wealth in Slavonija afterwards. No government could confiscate their brains. Their intelligence was, in fact, the real family treasure. There were no obstacles for people who wanted to work. They were smart enough to get out there and find some work to earn enough money to purchase new properties.

I recall our patch of land in Slavonija. As a child, I often visited there and I grew to love it. Now, this property is gone. We weren't even able to visit our grandfather's grave because it was now in Croatian territory, from which Serbs had been expelled. I knew my family's history in Slavonija well, but I don't know anything at all about my mother's side of the family from Lika. I would have liked to find out more, but I was frightened to do so. Why was my family reticent about its past? What were they hiding?

My maternal grandfather had been imprisoned in Croatia. He was released sometime after I was born. Not long after his release from prison, he was found dead. My family believed that he had been murdered. He was sent home in a sealed tin coffin, so they couldn't tell whether it really was his body that was con-

---

18. *Eighth Offensive*, Yugoslav Communist historiography uses the term "Seven Offensives" to designate military operations undertaken during WWII by the Partizans against the Axis powers. For this reason, Tito referred to the alleged return of refugees to their homes after WWII as the Eight Offensive.

cealed inside. After that, members of this branch of the family went their separate ways. One by one, they either moved to Serbia or went abroad. Members of my mother's family came to stay at my parents' house in Belgrade for longer or shorter periods of time until they were able to get back on their feet. One aunt went to live in France; one of my uncles, after years of wandering, finally ended up in Canada. The three remaining uncles and my other aunt stayed in Serbia. We enjoyed harmonious familial relations and we helped each other. Through hard work, they managed to earn enough so that they were able to live comfortably. My grandmother lived to an advanced old age, yet she was still haunted by memories of WWII. She, nevertheless, died satisfied because she knew that her children were able to stand on their own two feet. She's buried in Serbia. All that she left me was a ring, an heirloom that was over a hundred years old. A Star of David graces the ring, with two smaller ones on either side. In the middle is a large diamond that still hasn't revealed all of its secrets. I seldom wore it, so I put the ring away in a jewelry box where it remained for a long time, all but forgotten.

Knin is different from Banija and Glina, where I had spent the winter and spring of 1993. The war lasted far too long in Knin. These long-suffering, depressed, and desperate people have become quarrelsome and impatient. I feel unstable here, too. We're all swimming against the current in the same whitewater rapids. I didn't know whether I will sink or swim, but it doesn't matter anymore. My conscience is tormented because I feel responsible for the fate of the people of Knin after Serbia betrayed them. Yet today I know that I'm responsible only for my own life and the lives of my children. Everything else is beyond my control and I have no influence over those events. My good intentions are not enough. I don't complain anymore because I can't change the world. But that doesn't mean that I stopped trying to do my best.

I used to be an idealist but I've become a realist. I used to love the sky and a garden in full bloom, but today I'm satisfied with a single cloud and the few flowers that I tend.

The Search for My Roots

Dr. Stojanac is in charge of the Medical Corps of the VII Dalmatian Division. He was banished from Rijeka, Croatia. He's a modest, quiet, and introverted man. One day, he and Marko took me on a tour of the surrounding area. It rained the whole morning, but when they pulled up in front of the hospital in their jalopy to pick me up, the clouds parted and the sky opened above us in all its clear profundity. We heard the melodies of birds along the serpentine road that unfolded before us. Everything was hushed. I asked my guides to show me Ervenik, a village where one of my friends from Smederevo was born. This is where his elderly parents still live. I wanted to visit them because I had to deliver cash that my friend had entrusted to me. The road is dry. There's no snow. Off the road, we see stones and a few dwarf trees with twisted, tangled branches. The soil here is barren. I see only rocks, stunted trees, and sun. An otherworldly atmosphere clings to the countryside. In order to survive in these severe conditions, a person has to develop special character traits. Often, the inhabitants are tough on the outside but gentle on the inside. This region is so poor that only those who were born here love it — and they are the ones who are willing to fight for it.

The engine groaned into low gear as we began the uphill climb. The Krka River Valley lay behind us. Soon we would be in Romići, a hamlet near Ervenik. It's the biggest village in the area around Knin. We drive slowly through the village and pass an open shop where I recognized someone who's sitting outside. It's a one-eyed man in a wheelchair, and when I catch a glimpse of his hands, I see that one is prosthetic. Both his legs are missing. A bottle of beer is standing beside his wheelchair, and from time to time he raises it to take a swig. Beer trickles down on his shirt, but he pays no attention to it. I ask Marko to slow down so that I can take a closer look at him.

Yep! That's him, alright! He's the patient who spat in my face a few years back when I was working at the hospital in Knin. Later, he was taken to Belgrade where he had several operations. The surgeons saved one of his eyes, so now he was able to see. In the hospital, he met a nurse who took an active role in his treatment and recovery. She put all her energy into motivating him to fight for himself. In the end, she even left her own family in order to devote herself to caring for him. This was something that I thought happened only in movies. But life had produced a better story than any film producer could have. Now they were living in this remote corner of Krajina. She married the one-eyed man who had lost both legs, and whose arm had been amputated, the man whose will to live she had restored.

I saw no reason to stop and say hello to him. He wouldn't have remembered me, anyway. I was just one of the many doctors who had attended him. But he reminded me of the unpleasant situations in which we doctors all too often find ourselves. We often can't restore to our patients the quality of life they once led, even though they expected it of us. Sometimes, we have to halt treatment if it might result in the patient's death. I'm just a doctor, so I may never usurp the right to make such life-and-death decisions. That's playing God. Once they have been discharged, our patients must take responsibility for the quality of their own lives. They are the ones who confer meaning upon it. So, it was a bittersweet moment: my patient is alive, but he's letting alcohol destroy his life.

A little further down the road, we parked the car and continued on foot along a narrow path which led to the house where the elderly couple we were looking for lived. Grandpa was eighty-six, and Grandma was eighty. There was no running water in the village. They collected rainwater in tanks. The door of the house was open, so we entered freely. Grandma was sitting in the kitchen, while Grampa was lying in bed because he was running a fever. I always travel with my doctor's bag and medicine. It's often necessary to help people who have no access to a physician. I examined him and it became clear that he had pneumonia. I gave him an injection of antibiotics and an infusion of electrolytes because he had neither eaten nor drunk anything since falling sick. I suggested that he go to the hospital where he could get further care, but he refused. He said that he wanted to die at home. Grandma promised to call a nurse from town to give him the injections I left.

The small house was so dirty that I simply couldn't leave without cleaning up. The least that the three of us could do was to tidy up the place and wash and clean everything that needed cleaning, so two doctors and a colonel rolled up their sleeves and went to work. Marko brought in rain water from the collection tank. Dr. Stojanac made a fire in the small wood-burning stove where he heated up some water. I gathered all the pots, pans, plates, glasses, and cups and washed them. Their house was passably clean after a couple of hours of scrubbing. The old woman went to the chicken coop to gather some eggs, and then she went to the stable to get some smoked meat. She also found some potatoes and onions. That was the meal she prepared for us. It's an old Serbian custom to offer the best food to guests. To have declined would have been an insult.

We made tea for Grampa and told him to drink it slowly. He cheered up a little because I brought news of his son and grandchildren in Smederevo.

I got choked up when I said good-bye. I hated the Croats who wanted to throw this wizened and infirm couple out of the only home they've ever known — simply because they were Serbs.

Why couldn't Grandma and Grampa live and die in their own home in their own country?

The road from Ervenik led to the Krupa Monastery. We followed a winding two-lane blacktop until it reached a summit from which we could see the Krupanj Plain as well as the river bisecting it. This valley is largely hidden, so the sudden appearance of this delicate, verdant plain nestled among gray mountains is a breathtaking sight. We were approaching a bridge when in the distance an ancient Orthodox monastery with gleaming white walls came into view.

Tsar Milutin built the Krupa Monastery in 1317. The Monastery still houses relics and valuable cultural artifacts despite having been subjected to frequent devastations over the course of its history. In the 1960s, frescoes painted in 1622 by Georgije Mitrofanović, a monk from Hilandar, were re-discovered in its church. Icons painted by Jovan Apak, who was trained in the Italo-Cretian school, were also kept in Krupa. The relics of St. Jerotej are also there, as well as his coffin from the Rmnja Monastery. And in the treasury, one can see three corporal cloths that had once belonged to different Patriarchs of Jerusalem. The Monastery archive has preserved twenty-two Turkish edicts, the most interesting of which refers to the order of protection of the Krka Monastery issued by Sultan Mustapha II.

We entered the Monastery with reverential awe. The church's frescoed walls were filled with icons. We lit candles for the fallen soldiers of Krajina as well as for the living. Two officers, dressed in camouflage fatigues, appeared in front of me. They bowed their heads in respectful silence.

The Church, which preserved the spiritual life of its people, and the Army, which defended the people's culture and material inheritance, were united here. Many times throughout history these two institutions found themselves at odds; today, however, the officers showed their respect for the spiritual values of those who had lived and died before us.

Marko, who was personally acquainted with the eighty-seven-year-old Dean, Father Pavle Kozlica, introduced us to the aged priest. According to Serbian custom, we bowed before Fr. Pavle as before a monarch, and we kissed his hand. Taking Fr. Pavle's poor hearing into consideration, Marko spoke loudly and distinctly. It turned out that Fr. Pavle knew Colonel Marko and Dr. Stojanac well. They explained to him whose granddaughter I was and why I had come. When Fr. Pavle understood who I was, he held out his arms and asked me to come closer so that he could see my face. Then he embraced me.

While his old hand was caressing my face, tears came to his eyes. He said:

"Your grandfather may now rest in peace. His blood, coursing through your veins, has brought you here, my daughter. He would have been proud of you. In his name, I am also proud of you. Blessed are those who have not forgotten their roots."

He told me that my late grandfather Lazar was a member of the Royal Yugoslav Army, then a member of the Chetnik Movement in the struggle against Fascism. He had saved the lives of more than three thousand people that the Ustaše had driven into the Krupa Monastery, to which they had then set fire. In these parts, it was necessary to protect even women and children from the Fascist Ustaše. Songs in the epic vein survive from that period, and some of them even mention my grandfather by name. The old priest spoke ardently of him, describing him as a hulky man who stood a full two meters tall, who had blond upright hair as if he were a Viking, and whose weathered features concealed a gentle and sympathetic soul within. The war had turned him into a soldier, a warrior who was still remembered for his bravery.

My grandmother Jeka (Jelena) also paid a price. The Ustaše arrested her several times and threatened her with execution unless she revealed her husband's as well as his fighters' whereabouts. My grandmother was just as brave as her husband — she never gave him up. She miraculously survived. Then a rumor spread that she possessed supernatural powers because she had eluded certain death. My grandmother always said that it was God's will that she survived — because she had lived righteously. She knew that the hour of her death had not yet come. She believed each of us has been fated to die at an appointed hour, so there was no reason to fear it beforehand.

I remember Grandfather Lazar, as well. He was patient with us grandchildren. He allowed us do many more things when we were on his property than other relatives did. I used to wake up early in the morning to feed the horses in the stable. Sometimes I ran ahead of him, but he was never angry with me and the horses never hurt me. He even made me a small pitchfork so that I could pitch them hay, and he made a small brush so that I could groom the horses' legs. I can still see their muscles contracting as I brush them down. He was always amused by the things I'd whisper to the horses as they gently nuzzled me.

I was redefining my darling little grandfather as a soldier, a war hero. The words of Fr. Pavle, who knew him when he was young, filled me with pride and confidence in the decisions I had made. I had acted upon an instinct that was deeper than common sense, so I disregarded all well-meaning advice. I couldn't stop myself. I simply had to come here. I had to get involved. But I have to admit that no matter how certain I was that I was doing the right thing, I also had certain shameful second thoughts. Perhaps my critics were right, after all. Did I have the right to leave my children in order to come here to treat other people's children? But now, after having heard about my grandfather, who lost his life precisely because of the courage he had shown during the war, the dark and confusing knot in my soul was finally untied.

After the war, Fr. Pavle continued, the Communists arrested my grandfather and sent him to prison. During the war, he had been an anti-Fascist, but after the war he became anti-Communist. Although the Communists had confiscated our family's property, my grandparents always managed to earn more, but Tito's government finally confiscated everything. My grandfather protested, and was subsequently arrested. My mother spoke of those difficult times. Members of the Yugoslav Communist Security Service stood watch at their gate to make sure that there was no smoke coming from their chimney because my grandparents were not even allowed to bake bread. The Communists were trying to starve them slowly to death. My grandmother lived in the Krupa area with her elderly parents and the seven-surviving of eleven children they had. They survived not only because my grandmother was a hard worker, but also because of the kindness of Croatian neighbors who secretly helped them. That was why my mother firmly believed there were no good or bad nations; instead, there were only good or bad people in each nation.

After we left the Monastery, we followed the road as it continued to wind its way upwards. Below, we saw a deep chasm. The higher we climbed, the less soil and vegetation we found. A rocky terrain spread out before us. We stopped at a bend in the road, where Marko pointed out the Kanjiža River, which flowed through a deep jagged crevice that it had carved into stone.

An eagle rose from the forbidding depths of the gorge and flew skywards. There were many caves and clefts in the mountainside where Serbs used to hide from the Fascists during World War II. The bones of Serbian civilians still lie among these stones. I wondered whether history was going to repeat itself. In Serbia, the Serbs settled high in the mountains to hide from the

Turks. Our history teacher used to ask us pupils about our ancestry. He believed that the descendants of families who dwelled in the mountains had the best chance of being true ethnic Serbs. The Turks practiced *le droit du seigneur*,[19] so those who hailed from lowland regions were more likely to have Turkish blood. This practice of disgracing the bride and the subsequent mixing of the genes led to suicides and revenge killings. It also forced people to change their names to conceal their identity.

By ascending Mt. Velebit, I came to understand that I too was made of sun and stone, of strength and endurance. These stones were a part of me. I was afraid of finding shameful roots; instead, I discovered that my roots were rock solid and warmed by sun. My cheeks took on a rosy hue. Marko gave me a sidelong glance and smiled. I was grateful to him for having brought me here.

We stopped in a very small village called Svonja — which was my grandmother's family name — to ask a man who was standing on the roadside where we might find the foundations of what was once my grandfather's house. We knew that it had been destroyed during WWII and that only the foundation remained. The man, whose name was Boško Svonja, was a talkative fellow and he invited us into his house. He obviously didn't often have visitors. It was wartime, but that didn't mean anything to him. He was accustomed to living frugally. In his solitude, he had everything he needed. A bottle of home-made wine, syrupy and nearly black, quickly appeared on the table.

He asked us who we were, and when we told him, he arose and bowed before me. He explained that members of noble fami-

---

19. *le droit du seigneur*, the right arrogated by a feudal lord to enjoy sexual relations with female subjects on their wedding night.

lies were greeted this way. He repeated the stories about my mother's family, their former wealth, and my grandfather's courage. Boško was in the Krupa Monastery when it had been set on fire by the Ustaše. My grandfather had saved his life too that day. Life was unjust, he said, to strong, honorable men. Boško remembered when my Grandfather Lazar was killed. The authorities sent him to prison out of sheer spite. There were many people who were jealous of his success. Boško said that he had a photograph of my grandfather in uniform with the Chetnik Commander Đujić.[20] He went to look for it.

Đujić once hid in my grandfather's house, where he had once christened an uncle of mine. While he was searching for the picture, he told us that it was dangerous to have such photographs because they could have — and still can — put one's life in danger, but he had kept it anyway. I was nervous as he searched the drawers of his simple cupboard. In the end, the photograph wasn't there. His wife must have hidden it, he said.

We heard the bleating of sheep in the yard. There, a wrinkled old woman was carrying a new-born lamb as she was leading her flock. She stopped before the house and lowered the lambkin to the ground. The umbilical cord was still dangling from its belly. Its tiny, shaggy body was trembling at its first encounter with the cruel world. It was trying to stand on its flimsy legs. The mother quickly trotted up and began licking the remaining blood and mucus from the newborn's body. The ewe was encouraging its tiny offspring, as if saying: *Don't be afraid! You are not alone in this world.*

---

20. *Đujić, Momčilo* (1907–1999) was a Serbian Orthodox priest who left the cloth to become a Chetnik commander in northern Dalmatia after the Independent State of Croatia was created during WWII.

Behind me, Boško was still talking about the past, as if the past here were somehow different from the past elsewhere.

Three kilometers further on, we came across another house, this one of obviously modern construction. Three huge shaggy dogs were lying in the yard. They arose lazily. One of them barked. Soon, a young man came out to greet us. He confirmed that this was the Veselinović household that we were looking for. These were my cousins four times removed. Marko explained who I was, but my cousin said that he already knew who I was and that he knew I was here in Krajina. His brother had visited the hospital almost four years ago, where I treated him. There were fifteen children in their family. I remember that during my childhood we used to send them our old clothes every summer. Fashion wasn't important here in the ravines of Velebit. To eke out a living from stones is an adventure unto itself. There were nine children living in the small, white house, which had few rooms, but it was immaculate. Six children had already married and moved out to start their own families.

Their mother also was a tall, bony, beautiful woman who had no wrinkles at all. I'm still amazed by how Mother Nature preserves some people from the outward signs of aging. This woman hadn't had an easy life, but there was no outward sign of it. Her house was in no sense poor. Everything was plain, clean, and in its place. The children stood in single file according to their height, and, smiling curiously, they shook hands with us politely. No one spoke before the mother did; no one interrupted her. The children didn't even whisper. She communicated with them by simply conveying a look. This atmosphere suited me because it reminded me of my own strict upbringing. We were surprised and impressed. Did families like this one really still exist? In Serbia, children walk all over their parents; they talk back; and they're always asking their parents to buy them something.

The children's clothing was neat and clean but patched here and there. I wondered where they got basic necessities, such as food and clothing, in this land of stone and sun. They didn't even have a vegetable garden. When Marko asked them directly how they managed to survive, the mother replied indirectly by saying that finding shoes for the boys was the biggest challenge. Some of them were tall and needed extra-large sizes, which were hard to find anywhere, not to mention finding them in war-torn Krajina. Marko promised to get shoes from the military warehouse. The mother added that they were always hungry, but that they had gotten were used to it. In fact, she said that it wasn't even worth mentioning because affluence had failed to produce decent human beings. Only poverty strengthens the spirit, she said, and it teaches us the real values of life. When people have everything, they stop struggling, and they start taking everything for granted. Life is a struggle, so those who forget how to fight lose in the end. She had not given birth to losers, she said. Her children were healthy and strong. They had no time to feel depressed. Only idlers suffer from depression.

We smiled politely as she shared her theories with us, but her experience had certainly given her insight into human nature. Here, in these trackless regions, people don't want anyone to feel sorry for them, but she did agree to meet Marko in Knin to pick up a sack of flour and some other basic necessities that the government was providing to civilians.

The eldest son, whom I met in the hospital, was now hiding in the mountains. He had protested injustices in the Army. The soldiers hadn't received their pay for months, so they couldn't send remittances to their families, who were in turn unable survive on their own. He had asked the Army for three to five liters of gasoline so that he could bring food to his family by moped. He had managed to save rations by being parsimonious, and he had also gotten other contributions of food from friends who were acquainted with his family's difficult situation. But the Army refused to help him out even though he was one of the hardest-working, most dependable, and bravest of soldiers. So, he reacted accordingly to the injustice he had perceived. He drove a tank to a mountain top where he siphoned off the fuel from the gas tank. Now his family had something to live on for a while, but then he went AWOL because he was going to be sent to the stockade. He was safe in these ravines dotted with caves, his mother said sadly. His family regularly brought him food. They left it in places that were known only to him.

This disastrous war was going to destroy Krajina, she continued. Marko listened and nodded silently. He was a member of the Army she was criticizing, but he wasn't getting rich off this war. He came from the same stock as she did. Since the war had begun, he made every effort to fight corruption and organized crime in Krajina. I almost lost my life because of it.

After we finished drinking coffee, this extraordinary family took us to the ruins of my grandfather's home. We could tell by its foundation that it had been a large house. Here, my mother was born. No one knew exactly when she was born because her birth records, along with those of many others, were destroyed by the Ustaše when they set fire to the Krupska Monastery.

After the war, when the children returned to school, many were already too old to attend elementary school. So their parents resorted to telling the authorities that the children were younger than they really were so that they could be enrolled. My mother fell into this category. The official documents that were issued to her after the war indicated that she was younger than she really was.

I picked up two stones from the foundation that were still warm from the setting sun. I imagined that perhaps my grandfather had once touched them. I was going to keep one and give the other to my mother, which would bring back memories of her alpine childhood.

* * * *

22. I Am Christened

On Monday, February 14, 1995, I was christened at the Krka Monastery along with two other catechumens — a young doctor from Gospić and a refugee now living in Belgrade whose god-mother was the pathologist in our hospital. This solemn ceremony of formal induction into the Orthodox Church was a momentous experience.

Great white clouds patterned the sunlight from a transparent blue sky. The Krka River Valley resonated with joy. It was not quite spring but everything was already green. The solid, white stone Monastery stood in majestic prominence. Centuries of serenity surrounded us. Peace reigned. These pillars upheld the continuity of Serbian spirituality.

The Monastery was built in the first half of the fourteenth century by Jelena, sister of Tsar Dušan. I had been brought up in a Communist family that did not acknowledge the Church. Later, when it became fashionable to be christened, I resisted because of the faddishness. It felt hypocritical. I'm a humanist and I'm well aware of my ignorance and shortcomings. Yes, there are more things in heaven and earth than I'm aware of. And perhaps they are things of a higher nature than we ordinary mortals are capable of understanding. That is why there was plenty of room in my heart and mind for God. My parents were honest people; they helped everyone who needed help. They did so to the detriment of their own interests as well as to those of our own small family. That was how I was raised: to respect the values expressed in the Ten Commandments as well as the Bible. What I was unable to accept, and what my parents found intolerable, was the institution of the Church — and its priests who preached

God's mercy but who practiced it only for those who could pay for it. Church authorities refused to bury those who hadn't been christened during the Communist era unless the family paid separately for a christening. They also charged for the burial, which made them look like hypocrites who were fleecing the public. Although it may have been justifiable to pay a debt to the Church, which had suffered from years of neglect, I did not quite understand why someone should owe the Church just for having been born. What did this have to do with God's mercy?

In any case, I was not christened and I remained diffident. Why should I trust a Church that had taken advantage of its despairing people? The Church had profited from their insecurity and fear by imposing itself as mediator that brokered relations between ordinary people and God. I believed in God, but I did not believe in the institution of the Church, which is comprised of priests who are just as human as I am. I'm ready to dedicate my life to God and to justice — but not to greed. I had a long discussion about my dilemma with Bishop Longin, who listened carefully to my reasons against being christened. Bishop Longin had grown up in Australia, and had gone on to obtain his Ph.D. at Oxford. He came back to this country where he had never lived to minister to its people in difficult times.

In Krajina, the Church did not charge for christenings; however, there was a fixed rate in Serbia. The Bishop told me that he knew my family, and that it would be an honor as well as his duty to christen me. We talked for hours, when all of a sudden I felt the need for certainty, so I made the commitment to stand by the side I had chosen. I decided to be christened because of Marko's support. Bishop Longin turned the ceremony into an unforgettable event.

Nenad Jakovljević from the Belgrade Opera joined the Theological Seminary's student choir to sing at our christening ceremony. The Monastery resonated with their voices, and the ethereal and deeply fulfilling sacred choral music uplifted me. Standing erect, I read with a resolute voice the biblical passages that Bishop Longin had selected for me. Next, I was bowing, and then I kneeled.

The Archpriest Milorad Lončar, who performed the christening, said:

"I'm deeply aware of the importance of this moment. It's not by chance that the three of you are doctors serving here, three Serbian women, and from now on three members of the Orthodox Church in one of its westernmost outposts, in a monastery founded generations ago by a great Serbian woman. We share a centuries-old destiny, which is to defend our spirituality alongside the soldiers who defend the land on which we walk."

After the ceremony, Marko and I took a walk along the river bank. He's a man born of these mountains. His lithe body moves rhythmically before me as we climb a narrow path. His outstretched hand points out the beauty of the valley. Then he pauses at the trunk of a blossoming almond tree. We caress the fissured bark of the slender trunk which is crowned by beautiful white flowers that will soon yield a nut. The almond tree sways in the soughing wind. We've been silent too long. There are many things we want to say to each other.

"I know you're afraid I'll get killed either by the Croats or by our Mafia. But I can't turn my back on my people. I've been training all my life for this moment. It's war. I swore an oath of loyalty, to uphold and defend the values of the Serbian people. This vow may not be broken.

"I may have lost everything I had in this war, but I will not lose my honor. I will only leave Krajina after the last man goes. My mother lives here, as do my relatives. I can't leave them at the mercy of the enemy."

I stand in awe of this man. He's right. He's the kind of soldier we need to have but so often don't. Do I love Colonel Marko

Vrcelj? Or am I in love with his role in the war and his uniform, all of which impart the trust and security that I so badly need? I don't know. Marko is going to stay here until the end of Krajina or until the end of his own life. I have to leave, and take my love with me.

The valley around the Krka Monastery is holy. Here, we can empty our heart of words. But just beyond this charming valley, a relentless war is gnawing at Krajina's bones.

23. Back in Serbia

March 1995.

Krajina's tragic condition had colonized my body, so I ended up suffering a nervous breakdown. I also suffered from a bleeding stomach ulcer. I could hardly walk. I spent one day on duty while I was delirious. I was on sick leave for more than a month. After I recovered, I collected medicine for the Army — and only for the Army — because they were held in contempt. I was going against the grain. I didn't want to help anyone else. If it weren't for the Army, Krajina would have disappeared long ago. No one understands that Krajina's small Army has been humiliated and brought to the threshold of human endurance.

After a few months, I was able to see things more clearly and I realized why Krajina had been defeated. I wasn't able to distinguish between those who were working for it and those who were working against it. Many took part in fighting simply because they thought they could pocket few thousand deutschemarks by plunder and theft. But they weren't ever going to get their homeland back after having spent those deutschemarks. Serbia was their sister, who had helped them and would help them again, but it wasn't their homeland. Sooner or later, they were going to understand this.

Dr. Nikolić, the Director of the Smederevo Hospital, was a kind-hearted man who sympathized with me — even during my violent emotional outbursts. He once again helped me collect medicine and he assured me that we could take anything we needed. But the Director of the Velika Plana Hospital thought differently. He asked me to sort out the forgotten medicine that had been languishing in storage for more than two years. By the time I finished the job, I was suffocating from the dust in the storage room. Then I learned that he had pulled a fast one on me! He told me to come with a big truck from Smederevo to take the supplies, but then he gave orders to give me only a fraction of the medicine I had sorted. If that small amount hadn't been indispensable to my colleagues in Glina, I would have left everything behind in disgust. But I got more than I could have imagined from the Smederevska Palanka Hospital. The Director and her pharmacist gave me everything on our want list. I believed for a long time that women were the better part of the world, and now I'm convinced of it.

Lieutenant Colonel G., the Chief Medical Officer in Krajina, with whom I had been coordinating the effort, was delighted. He said:

"My God, Dr. Mitić, I've never seen anything like this! They told me that no one was going to help us. It's not true. You should have seen the civic leaders in Smederevo. They ran after our trucks to wish the drivers a safe journey. You told me Smederevo had a high rate of mobilization — about 140 wounded, 40 killed. I know the town led the fight for the right of the veterans of this war to receive apartments, as well as for support to be given to the children of those who had been killed in action. Is this your doing, Doctor, or are the people of Smederevo just naturally generous?"

"I can't say," I replied. "I couldn't get anything they weren't willing to give."

Colonel G. was now gone. I don't mind that the driver and I have to lift and load those critical supplies onto the truck ourselves. My so-called 'gentlemen' colleagues pass us by, averting their eyes as I lift one huge box after another. When we arrive in Krajina, one of the men unloading the shipment has the gall to demand a hundred dinars per hour for overtime. They're Serbs, to boot! Love for one's country is disintegrating, rotting away from the inside out.

* * * *

The VMA Director sent two cars to pick up all the doctors from Krajina who were doing residencies in Serbia. They planned to go to Krajina through the only free point of entry in the north. The Director passed over those who were known to have been disloyal.

A team of doctors from the VMA left for Krajina on Sunday morning, but the VMA lost contact with them. I asked if they needed me. I was ready to go.

"No, it won't be necessary. There'll be enough of us," said Dr. Srđan, Head of Anesthesiology. "We'll manage! Thanks!"

That single sentence saved my life. I stayed home. I didn't witness the fall of Krajina.

I'm wondering as I listen to the news: *How can the announcers read this news report with such calm and dispassionate voices?* Grahovo and Glamoč have fallen. Dinara has been conquered. I'm not very good at geography, but one thing is clear: if you take three sides, you will then take the fourth easily. Knin had already been cut off from the Republika Srpska. How are those doctors supposed to get there? Who's going to take care of the wounded? There are only sixty doctors in the whole of Krajina, including pharmacists. The others have already fled to Serbia.

I have another personal reason for agonizing over Krajina's fate. It has been a while since I've heard Marko's reassuring voice, which always calms me down. Then I hear his voice in my mind's ear: *The Ustaše will never defeat Krajina in an armed conflict, Sarah. Krajina and I are doing well.... Don't you cry. You don't cry for the living.*

After that, I calm down and go to sleep, happy to suppose that he's alive, but I don't know what tomorrow may bring, so I don't dare think about it any longer.

At five o'clock in the morning on August 5, 1995, Croatian forces launch a surprise attack against Krajina, and set all its towns and villages ablaze. At ten minutes past six, I listen to General Mrkšić's announcement on the radio: "The Army is stationed in reserve positions. The people have been evacuated. We support our soldiers."

Then there's a long pause. I tune into other radio stations. Then I turn on the television. Nothing. Silence! I scream in the bathroom so as to not awaken my brother and sister-in-law.

Then Radio Free Europe announces: "Knin has fallen. The Croats are marching triumphantly into town."

I lay in bed agonizing. Where are those whom I love? Are they alive? Is Marko alive? Once I get over my initial uncontrolled emotions, I analyze what I've heard. An irrational hope arises that it isn't true. I'll never believe that they're dead. Marko's alive. Alive!

The telephone starts ringing nonstop. Marko's sister and I exchange our last optimistic hopes. What has happened to our families? What has happened to the old men and the children? When I walk down the streets, I hate every Serbian face I see because they didn't go to Krajina to help. O, Serbia, you should be ashamed! I don't care whether the so-called protectors of Serbia have heard me or whether they'll pack me off to prison. Prison can't possibly be as bad as the pain I now feel.

I question numerous people who are in the know: can the people of Krajina defend themselves? I get the same answer over and over again: "No! Krajina doesn't have an Army. The Army of Krajina is its people."

A few officers don't make an Army. To tell the truth, able-bodied men of draft age are more interested in obtaining perquisites from the new authorities than they are in defending their country. The Americans are training and arming the Ustaše. The war has lasted for five years, so men from Dalmatia, and especially from Knin, are keen on avoiding mobilization. There are one hundred thousand men from Knin, all eligible for the draft, who are now in Belgrade. And they were expecting my brother, who was born in Belgrade, to defend their native territory!

The Serbs are winning another victory in the battle against their own interests.

In these tragic moments, I wish I knew much less than I do; saw much less than I did. Then I would be able to blame Milošević and get the rancor out of my system. But I can't. I'm certain that Milošević is not the only one to blame. Krajina is now defended only by those whom Krajina had humiliated the most: the JNA soldiers who chose to remain. God save us!

I count my reasons for staying in Smederevo. In spite of everything, I'm tempted go to Krajina again. But what would happen to my children if I went away again? In the past, my desire to help people was greater than my fear of death. Now, the fact that I was needed at home outweighed my impulse to go.

Finally, the telephone rings and I hear his warm voice saying: *Hello…!*

Marko's alive!

"Are you alright? Where's your family? Talk to me!" I say, the words tumbling out.

"Am I alright? Can't say. I didn't know there was anything the matter with me to begin with."

I want to hit him for kidding around with me at a time like this.

"My family's okay. They're on their way to Banja Luka. They'll arrive in Serbia in a few days. Sarah, the people are alive! As long as they're alive, don't grieve for Krajina! Both Krajina and I are alive. A living man can go to prison and still come out alive...."

On Monday, I go to Belgrade to meet colleagues from the hospital in Knin who got out alive. We embrace tearfully. We tacitly acknowledge that something vile has become part of us. We're ashamed to be alive!

Jelena is lying helpless on the floor. She's wailing.

"I want Krajina back! I want my hospital back! I want to live near my father's grave. I don't know what I'm doing here. I don't want this!"

Others likewise suffer. Some are sobbing; others are speechless with shock. Some need to talk about the details; others, who've had enough, just want to vanish from the face of the earth. One story follows another. They're seething with misery and rage. Information is sketchy. Everyone has their own version of events, and they're all drawing their own conclusions.

The telephone is ringing nonstop with calls from Banja Luka, Australia, Switzerland, Loznica, Požega, and Sremska Rača. I'm glad to be with people who love Krajina. I'm glad they're still alive. Everything else can wait. The living call the living to tell them they're still alive. I want know the whole story. How did the siege start? Did they know it was coming? What happened to the Army? But they never manage to piece it together. I realize that I'm not making any sense. Nor is anyone else.

Initially, they're reluctant to speak. They're anxious and exhausted. The men are chain smoking. Their hands tremble. No one can eat anything. The last few days, they didn't even leave the hospital. They were tending to wounded soldiers from Strmice, Grahovo, and other nearby areas. Even the night before the bombardment, no one had a clue that Knin was going to fall. They say a group of soldiers made it through from Dinara to visit a seriously wounded officer who was in Intensive Care. These soldiers said that the Ustaše were already in Igla and that they were on their way to Crvena Zemlja. No one could believe it because that meant the end of Knin. No one wanted to scare off the staff, but the wounded officer defended his men. If they said the enemy had reached Igla, then their information was credible. All seemed lost. A host of questions quickly arose. How long could the Army defend Knin? Was Serbia going to send reinforcements? Or was Serbia abandoning Krajina? Then — horrified silence.

They said a crescent moon appeared in the dark sky above Mt. Promine. First, it was bright yellow, and then right before their very eyes the crescent moon began changing color as a rainbow does from yellow to orange and then, starting from the lower horn, to blood red: A Blood Moon over Krajina.

Some recall poems about the Battle of Kosovo that describe how the sky shed tears for the Serbs before the battle. Is this happening again? Two hours later, the bombardment of Knin began. Grenades exploded near the hospital. The shelling was deafening. Some level-headed members of the hospital staff prepared to evacuate. They took seriously injured patients down to the first floor, where military helicopters were landing between mortar rounds. Many wounded soldiers panicked and began pulling out their chest tubes. In the ensuing chaos, the doctors and nurses tried to quiet them down and keep their tubes in place. Sometimes as many as ten, at other times as few as three, wounded soldiers could be evacuated by helicopter at any one time, depending on how much time the pilots had. They couldn't really land, so they took in the wounded as the helicopter was hovering. Once again, these courageous pilots were bearing the brunt of the war.

This reminds me of my friend Marica, whose brother is a helicopter pilot. He doesn't even have his own apartment, so he has to rent one for his family in Montenegro. He and other pilots are risking their lives while there are many officers from Krajina who are sitting out the war in comfortable Belgrade apartments, the likes of which those who are really doing the fighting would never have.

As a newly minted patriotic Serb, I find the following story unacceptable. But I'm of two minds as a human being and as a doctor, so I didn't know what to make of it. Some members of the hospital staff were making urgent preparations for evacuation. They were moving equipment and patients downstairs; others, however, were watching calmly from the sidelines.

"Where are you going?" the Head of the Anesthesiology Department, who was also Krajina's Deputy Minister of Health, was reported to have asked. "Why are you panicking? We're doctors. Nothing's going to happen to us. This is just scaremongering. The Croats are civilized people. They're not going to harm us. We're going to stay right here. We have nowhere to go. Serbs or Croats, we were born here and this is where we're going to stay. So calm down and get ready to meet the leadership of the new government."

It's difficult for me to hear this story. He's a man who had saved a thousand Serbian lives during the war. I think about conversations we had. I admire him as a physician and as an intellectual, but now I'm stunned. Some said it was the right thing to do. He was trying to calm everyone down. And even I, on the one hand, do feel differently as a human being than I do, on the other, as a doctor. When the chaos began, he sent home the only technician who was a volunteer from the VMA. A week ago, he told me not to come. But wasn't I needed, after all? Can anyone say, without a shadow of a doubt, that he was right? Another anesthesiologist stayed, as well, and two nurse-anesthetists. Dr. Jovan, heartbroken with disbelief, remained lying in his room under the influence of sedatives and alcohol. He also refused to leave Knin.

He kept repeating to himself: "Knin is not going to fall. Serbia will never allow Knin and Krajina to fall."

There were a thousand dilemmas but only two choices: either to leave with the patients who could be moved or to stay with the hospital-bound patients and the staff members who had decided to await the arrival of the Croats.

It's difficult to listen to all this. I understand that it can be seen as a choice between the lesser of two evils. People have the right to decide for themselves. Some stayed; others left with a heavy heart. One and all faced an uncertain fate. The staff members who chose to stay prepared welcome speeches for their new masters. They had to be careful not to make a slip in their accent. It was certain that this "promising new democratic" government wasn't going to tolerate people speaking the Ekavian dialect, the standard Serbian dialect that had become widespread in Krajina since the war began. They were also going to ban the use of the Cyrillic alphabet, which had not even been used there until the war began.

The group of staff members I spoke with told me that they had fled the hospital in a panic only to discover that there were neither buses — nor even a single available ambulance — to evacuate patients. The vehicles had disappeared. People who left quickly didn't have the time for second thoughts. Doctors, nurses, and staff still dressed in their green and white scrubs and clogs began to flee. The remaining patients stayed with the doctors and nurses who had decided not to leave.

Those who were fleeing cursed the day they were born. How could they have been such cowards as to leave their patients behind? They didn't believe that the impending arrival of the "representatives of democracy" was going to bode well for them. When I was in Knin during the bombardments in 1991, I remembered the chaos caused by the bombs that struck during the air raids. The patients told us to escape and to leave them with weapons so that they could kill one more Ustaše before they themselves died. Now I don't even dare imagine the bombs that were falling on Knin after it had been surrounded. No one issued an order to retreat; people simply up and left. Panic-stricken doctors fled with as many bandages and syringes as they could stuff in their pockets, along with a lethal dose of drugs to kill themselves if they were captured. Chaos reigned on all the routes leaving Knin. A stampeding column of human beings was crushing everything in its path.

UNPROFOR soldiers, I am told, were smirking icily as they stood silently by and did nothing. Doctors implored these soldiers to deploy armored vehicles and to use megaphones to rescue members of the hospital staff who were still at home and who may not have known of what was happening. Not one UNPROFOR soldier was willing to do this. It wasn't their war; it wasn't going to be their defeat; and it wasn't going to be their fault if anyone got killed. But one Russian soldier, remembered only as Andrei, agreed to help. He went and got three staff members in his personnel carrier, but he was unwilling to go back for anyone else. Shells were hitting streets and buildings. One column of desperate people was fleeing uphill on foot where they were greeted by bombs — so they changed direction.

Doctors and military reservists were evacuating their families. These people were the only soldiers the Krajina Army had. It was the fighting force that was supposed to defend Krajina. The national Army, after having been cut to minimum numbers, heroically resisted the attacks and protected the people. Srb and Martinbrod were the last two escape routes left on Knin's perimeter.

A rumor spread in the refugee column: *Milan Martić committed suicide in his office.* They nodded gravely with approval. *For once in his life, he did something honorable,* they said. But he hadn't actually committed suicide. The International Criminal Tribunal in The Hague indicted him later.

Somewhere near Petrovac, the police called for doctors and medical personnel from the column. The Bosnian doctors had deserted the hospital. One surgeon managed to muster a medical team from the Knin refugees right in the street. They began working immediately even though they were exhausted and distraught. One medical student, an intern who was specializing in anesthesia, couldn't have had a tougher assignment than assembling and prepping an anesthetic machine that she was seeing for the first time in her life. They performed four operations under appalling conditions. During a break, they were given dry bread.

From that moment on, it was each man for himself. People coped as well as they could in conditions of utter chaos. Throughout Bosnia, which had its own problems, columns of refugees were wandering down roads that led to salvation in Banja Luka. One group arrived at a border crossing with Serbia in a jalopy that had neither a windshield nor a rear window. The car was falling apart as they were driving it. They were pale with shock and covered with blood and dust. After crossing the border into Serbia, each went his own way. At first, they were only interested in saving their own lives. Now, as I'm listening to them, I'm not even sure whether their own lives were still important to them. They spoke to each other on the phone for days on end.

A doctor from Banja Luka phones to inform us that the TV news aired a report about the arrival of Croatian troops at the Knin Hospital. He caught a glimpse of the faces of Dr. Savo J., Dr. Rajić and Dr. Jovan on screen. Their faces were swollen and bruised. There were nurses who stayed, as well: Nurse Duška, a wonderful, hardworking, head anesthetist from Biskupija; Nurse Goca; and Nurse Neda who was known to have collaborated with Ustaše. On that same Croatian news broadcast, the announcer said that the Serbs were dirty and that their hospital was filthy, too. That hospital was cleaner than all the hospitals I've worked at in Serbia! And, according to my colleagues, it was cleaner than 90% of Croatian hospitals. Why do they always have to lie about every little thing?

The lives of many captured and wounded Croatian soldiers had been saved in that hospital, but who could have reasonably expected the victors to conduct themselves in a dignified manner toward the defeated? Panic-stricken people say all sorts of things which can't always be believed. My question is simple: *Why did all this have to happen at all? Why did this war start in the first place?*

I can't take it anymore. I lie motionless in bed. I can't eat much less open my mouth. If I get an unexpected phone call, I roar angrily into the receiver. I don't care about anything anymore. I want to lie down and sleep. On Saturday, I was awakened from a feverish sleep by the ringing telephone. My heart leapt. He's alive! Suddenly, the room was full of light. My life force rushed into my ears from the forgotten recesses of my body so I could hear him better.

"I'll be there in an hour. I'm waiting for the transport from Belgrade."

I did now in one hour all the things that I hadn't been able to do for days. I prepared dinner. I tried to think of everything he might need. I didn't know what his state of mind would be when I saw him. It didn't matter just as long as he was alive! When the bell rang, I opened the door with a trembling hand. I didn't even look into his eyes when I threw my arms around his neck. I was afraid to see the void left by the fall of Krajina.

He threw his duffle bag on the floor and said: "Sarah, I've got nothing left."

I was happy that he had come back alive, but I knew that he needed Krajina. I was thinking of all the women waiting for their husbands, brothers, and fathers who had gone to fight, who may return wounded or who will never return. I was one of the lucky ones.

"You've still got your head on your shoulders and you can walk from point A to point B. I don't need anything else. Welcome home!"

The search for loved ones from Krajina continued for days afterward. Fifty members of my family arrived from Golubić, Obrovac, and Gračac. I took care of those from Banija and Kordun. O my God, there were so many people! They're alive, but what was going to happen a month from now?

The Commissariat for Refugees is running smoothly. They work tirelessly to help us. We get the information we need quickly, and they're kind. I wonder where they get the patience to deal with all of us who are looking for loved ones.

Marko and I travel around Serbia to look for familiar faces. It's in a motel near Ruma in Vojvodina in Northern Serbia where I run into Nurse Mirina, my friend from Banija, who has a fiery and uncontrollable temperament. We scream when we recognized each other and we run into each other's arms. She hasn't changed a bit. Even in Banija, Mirina's optimism and energy stand out. I haven't seen her since 1993. I ask her how people in Banija reacted to my depictions of them in my Journal. She tells me some were unhappy about it; nevertheless, Mirina defended me by saying that I hadn't invented either my own or anyone else's misfortunes; that I bore witness to the tragic history of a wonderful, humane people; and that they should have given some thought to what kind of people they are before they discovered my portrayal of them.

We spot a broken down car with registration plates from Glina parked in front of another motel. There I found a group of people whom I knew. They gathered around tables out on the motel's terrace. They're silent, pale, and gaunt. Many are in mourning because many people have been killed. I didn't know how to approach the survivors. I yearn to help them, but I can't. I feel that I let them down somehow. It's my personal nightmare.

Dragica, the Head Surgical Nurse, stands by the door. I look for the old glitter and audacity that once resided in her beautiful blue eyes. For me, she's still the same cheerful, courageous nurse from Glina. Even so, her evident misery breaks my heart. I know that her younger daughter, who's still in elementary school, drove a tractor from Glina to Ruma. The girl's sneakers had been torn to shreds from pressing the brake pedal so often during the long journey. I can't let my memories of Dragica's vivacity fade into the drab hopelessness of a ramshackle motel. I hear that my beautiful nurse Zeljka, now pale and suffering from depression, has a baby that's only fifteen days old.

We find Krčo and his wife Nada, a nurse, their two children, and his elderly mother in one of the motel rooms. Krčo had been wounded in the chest, leg, and both arms during a firefight near Vojna in Banija. He spent two days laying half-dead where he had fallen. The Muslims deliberately ignored him and left him to die in agony. They wouldn't even put him out of his misery with a *coup de grâce*. He drank the morning dew, and thanks to the beneficial effects of worms that had infested his wounds, he didn't get sepsis. (It's a well-known phenomenon that worms have an anti-inflammatory effect on wounds.) When they found him, he was taken to the Glina hospital. Nada was just as happy as if he had been reborn. Nurse Mirina tells me how she took the worms out of his open chest. He left everything behind in the rolling hills of his native Banija. Now he tells me he has nothing, but Nada quickly interjects that he has everything because he was still alive.

Krčo was rescued on September 2, 1994, which is a new holiday that celebrates our continued survival, we say joking with Krčo. But he's depressed. He's concerned about his elderly mother.

After I return home, I nearly faint from the shock of meeting all these people in a dreary motel, people whose lives have been ruined. I just can't write about them anymore. Yet I know that these pages may mean one thing today, but tomorrow they will stand as factual testimony to this moment in history.

Wherever I may go, my homeland will come with me. My family is all I have, and I'll never get attached to anything else. If, by chance, I were to settle in Bulgaria, then I'd make it my home. I wouldn't grieve for lost territory or material possessions. But what is going to happen to these children who are now growing up? What kind of an example are we going to set for them if we surrender to pain and suffering?

I searched for others who were scattered throughout Serbia. They were hoping to find work in hospitals. Their experience in Glina made them invaluable.

I found Dara in Čačak. Her husband Đuro had suffered a heart attack. That gentle, brave, heartbroken man couldn't reconcile himself to what had happened. I hoped that he would get well, and that Dara would get a job as an anesthesiologist in Serbia.

I neither watch television nor read the newspapers. I'm sickened by the so-called humanitarianism that's nothing more than a tepid glass of milk served with a smile. What these unfortunate people need is jobs. If they produced enough to make a living on the barren soil of Krajina, then imagine what wonders they could do with the fertile land in Serbia?

Two or three years ago, I met people in Krajina who had nothing but contempt for Serbia. They called it the country of pepper and plum growers back then, but now Serbia has opened its bosom to embrace those who needed help. Serbia never betrayed anyone. Serbians may break their promises on occasion, they may even be unfaithful to themselves, but Serbia never has and never will. This is the Serbia that I love and this is the Serbia that steps forward now, far away from newspaper articles and television cameras. This is the Serbia that produced sacks of flour that my neighbor Jelica handed out to refugees.

24. The Fall of Krajina

It's the end of summer 1995. Autumn is approaching. Ripening crops are ready for harvest. Perhaps an autumn peace will arrive.

Columns of refugees are still struggling to reach Serbia. Marko and I keep searching for members of our families from Krajina in refugee centers throughout Serbia. The situation became tense when a phone call from Belgrade surprised us. Vanja Bulić, the journalist from the weekly magazine *Duga* (Rainbow), who had published excerpts from my War Journal and who had interviewed me on his program *Crni biseri* (Black Pearls), called to ask if I would write something for their magazine. My article would have been just another commentary, among many others, on the fall of Krajina. I had neither the time nor the desire to write it. I could barely cope with the pain that kept growing with each passing day, and I feared that it might soon overwhelm me and leave me bereft of the powers of reasoning and common sense. I'm demoralized and disoriented. I don't like this new world, and I don't like the Serbian authorities. One and all have disappointed me because they've not only been unfaithful to their purported humanitarianism but also disloyal to their own people. How can I be expected to write honestly in this state of mind? And I'm not going to lie. The columns of refugees aren't going to permit any lies to be told about their situation. Friends keep arriving with the latest news. An orthopedist from Knin was trapped with his wife and sick child somewhere near Jagodina in a weekend cottage in the mountains that had no running water. They were without their possessions. He was going around crazy-angry bouncing off of trees. I can see his once laughing face in my mind's eye. He was always willing to work. His daughter has cerebral palsy. What's going to happen to them? It's hard enough for people who are healthy, but it's even worse for the sick and the handicapped.

I am tormented by the images of people who have been driven from their homes in Krajina and who have been forced to live in refugee camps or temporary accommodations in war-weary Serbia.

I ask the Director of the Smederevo Hospital to employ our colleagues from Krajina. They're good doctors. They need jobs for their physical as well as emotional rehabilitation. The hospital needs specialists, and this is a great opportunity to fill those spots. The benefits are obvious: the hospital gets the trained specialists it needs, and the refugees get a chance to start a new life. This would be a much better outcome than their receiving unemployment benefits that Serbia can't afford to pay, anyway.

But the Director gives me a helpless look. He shows me a document from the Ministry of Health stating they're not allowed to employ medical personnel from Krajina. They have to return to the places where they came from. I can't believe it! What kind of a policy is this? What are their standards of humanity, compassion — dignity?

Vanja Bulić calls me again and insists that I voice my opinion publicly. I'm of two minds about whether to accept his offer. First of all, who am I to comment on the matter? Marko, who's standing next to me, says in a low voice:

"She is coming around, Vanja. She's been despairing, but she's coming around. She can't remain silent and she won't. You and I know it. This country is lucky to have people who will speak up in protest. What happened in Krajina left people speechless, but the truth has to come out. Sarah's coming around. She knows this is bigger than she is."

Marko received orders to follow the rest of the Army to Bosnia. They are going to regroup and reform the Army of the Republic of Krajina. From there, they are supposed to make plans to return to Krajina. This is utter nonsense! How are a few Serbian officers going to win against the well-organized Croatian Army that has U.S. backing?

Marko went to Bosnia.

One day, in the *Braća Karić* studios where *Crni biseri* was broadcast, I was waiting my turn to go on air. I was trying to catch my breath after the three-hour journey from Smederevo to Belgrade, which turned out to be a real adventure. Municipal transportation in Belgrade has been curtailed because of a shortage of operable buses. Years of sanctions have prevented the city from obtaining spare parts. Things aren't collapsing slowly; they're getting visibly worse by the day. Public transportation is operating over and above its capacity. There is a gasoline shortage. And there is no funding available for new buses, trams or trains. So, sweaty, nervous, and aggravated passengers end up being packed like sardines into the few remaining buses that are running.

When my turn finally came to go on air, I took a seat across from Vanja and I began telling my story. Before long, I simply broke down in tears. I wasn't ashamed, but I was ashamed of the Ministry of Health, which wasn't allowing medical personnel from Krajina to work in Serbia. The people who had stayed in Krajina for five years and had survived the horrors of war were now being left out in the cold. I came to beg for help. The doctors, nurses, and technicians didn't want charity. They need employment, respect, and acceptance in our community. It's our duty to restore their sense of human dignity.

Persecution

The television broadcast unleashes a strong public reaction which keeps growing much like the concentric rings that arise when a stone is tossed into still waters. Letters of support begin arriving. They're simply addressed with my name: Sarah Z. Mitić, Smederevo. People call me on the phone and express their support, which means a great deal. I'm confused because I'm used to criticism. But soon scorn and persecution rear their ugly heads. A group of doctors from the Smederevo Hospital staff wants me fired!

It's painful to be shunned by my fellow staff members. Have my colleagues become so indifferent to reality? I can't even remember anymore what I said during the broadcast. I remember only the tears. The only thing I want is justice and fair treatment for the medical personnel from Krajina. They have nowhere else to go!

I try to work off my tension by jogging ten kilometers every day through the hills lined by grapevines that lie just outside Smederevo. I have to endure. What I'm experiencing is negligible compared to what people from Krajina had to endure. This isn't personal tragedy — it's a national tragedy.

The pressure comes in waves: at one moment it's unbearable; the next it seems to abate. "This too will pass one day. Even the longest day must end," I keep repeating to myself as I run kilometer after kilometer through the hills. The wind and the sun are refreshing.

I endured a six-month boycott against me at the hospital by the time the storm finally subsided. The Hospital Director hired twelve medical personnel from Krajina, among them an orthopedist from Knin and his wife, who's also a doctor. Our old proverb holds true: *Only in adversity does heroism appear.*

The Disabled Veterans from Krajina
— The Warriors Whose Wounds Will Never Heal

Permanently disabled veterans are arriving along with the refugees. About a hundred and eighty are being accommodated in the Rudo Rehabilitation Center. The conditions are overcrowded and dreadful. The Center used to have high standards which are now rapidly deteriorating because it hasn't been funded since the war began. The Center accommodates chiefly disabled civilians, men and women who have lost arms, legs or both, either in Krajina or in Bosnia. Here they are learning how to function with their disabilities as well as they can while waiting for prostheses. They quickly formed, with the support of friends, an association called "Good Will" which is led by Dušan, a sculptor and stonemason from Krajina. A bomb had blown his legs off, along with an arm and an eye. He's crippled for life but he remains of sound mind and he has a phenomenal will to live. He continues to paint. On the one hand, he's expending creative energy, which rescues him from boredom; but on the other hand, it's a constant reminder of all the things he can no longer do. He finds it difficult to concentrate on the things that he *can* do. For many of the disabled, alcohol has become a reliable source of comfort and relief. Inebriation deludes them into imagining that they're happy, yet they know the truth down deep inside. No drunk was ever happy, and such unhappiness can clearly be discerned in Dušan. His face expresses pain and despair. There are a number of humanitarian organizations that are trying to help these people, but nothing constructive is being done for their long-term management.

The disabled have to make frequent hospital visits for treatment as well as for the preparation for prostheses. It's not easy to find available spots for them in hospitals, and even when one is found, the patients themselves are often disruptive and they cause other problems. One night, an orthopedist called me. He had only reluctantly agreed to admit Dušan to the hospital to provide surgical treatment for his truncated limbs.

Now the orthopedist was shouting at me over the phone: "Come right now and get this idiot of yours out of here!"

"What did he do?" I asked cautiously.

"It would be easier to tell you what he hasn't done! The list would be a helluva lot shorter! He's nuts! Get him out here! This is an Orthopedic Ward — not an insane asylum. Take him to the Psycho Ward ... and find a spot for me, too!"

When I arrived, I found a grotesque but humorous scene. Someone had given Dušan a bottle of brandy, so he got loaded, and then the other patients in the room joined him and they got tanked, too. Now they were singing like the drunken crew of a pirate ship. They had untied their bandages and thrown them on the floor. The red stumps of their limbs stared at me like eyes without sight. The patients were grinning. Their faces were flushed. I understood the doctor, but I understood Dušan, too. I had to awaken a friend in the middle of the night and ask him to come pick Dušan up and take him back to the Rudo Center. We never mentioned this episode again. There were many such incidents, but any further elaboration would be pointless.

After having completed a rehabilitation course, the greatest problem facing these permanently disabled patients is accommodations. Their families are refugees just as they are, and they're scattered throughout Serbia in refugee camps. In some places, a hundred people are sleeping in the same room. That's why these patients are doomed to stay at the Rudo Center, where they have little or no contact with their families.

Those of us who take an active role in their rehabilitation do visit the patients, and we do the best we can to alleviate their suffering. We encourage them to write and to paint. In other words, we don't want them sitting around all day long staring at a wall or getting drunk. Their minds have to be occupied. Otherwise, the overwhelming awareness of their grim reality can lead to insanity. Well-known actors come and perform for them. In one particularly absurd proposal, a few American companies offered to donate electronic prostheses on the condition that the patients travel to company-owned laboratories and participate in experiments. It was horrible. First the Americans turn them into war invalids, and now they want to conduct experiments on them!

It's a sad sight to behold the invalids protesting: "Hitler did that, too!" they shout.

Serbia will never be able to offer them prostheses, and without them, they'll remain immobilized and bed-ridden. I can't think straight any more. It's too painful. And what will happen if they refuse? The people who made these prostheses were not likely to have been the ones who were dropping bombs on them. They, perhaps, don't even know anything about this war. They may not even have the faintest idea of where Yugoslavia is.

I give the guys a little time to vent their fury, then I try to persuade them to accept the offer, after all. I do manage to persuade a few.

Much later, I met them at a party that was held on their behalf. I was moved to tears when one of them asked me to dance. A handsome young man, missing a shoulder and an arm, now held my hand with a prosthesis that was so perfectly made that it looked like a real hand. To look at him, no one would have suspected that he had prosthesis. Dressed in suits, they looked like themselves before the war. A former auto mechanic got prostheses for both his lower legs and he was able to dance the *kolo* — the Serbian folk dance performed in a circle while holding hands. I shed tears of joy. God, how I cried that evening!

The auto mechanic returned to his job and started making a living again. The prostheses had restored his former self-reliance. An engineer who had lost a leg made a parachute jump with his prosthetic leg, which withstood the test. For many of these people, prostheses had successfully replaced lost limbs, while poetry, prose, and painting filled the emptiness in their souls. Most difficult of all is the patient's recovery from shock.

Several books have been written about the intellectual and creative achievements of our disabled veterans. I met many wonderful people during this period. For very practical reasons, some of them were the members of SPS (Socialist Party of Serbia), which was how they were able to save their own lives and social positions. This enabled them to be of even greater help to other disabled veterans. They advised me to do the same in order to protect myself from persecution. A growing number of acquaintances had suggested the same idea. As they say: *If you can't beat 'em, join 'em.* My own life was becoming unbearable because I was then barely able to endure the constant attacks to which I was subjected. I lived for my children, so, for their sake, I had no right to reject well intentioned advice, but the real question was whether or not the party would want me now.

In order to help the disabled vets, I participated in conferences to raise donations from Serbs who were living abroad. Those who were willing to make donations couldn't be certain that the financial support they intended to provide was going to go into the right hands or whether it was going to be absorbed by some for-profit business. They obviously didn't want to throw money down a black hole. Their initial idealism vanished quickly. This approach was difficult to implement and, in the end, the effort was unsuccessful.

We were in the Hotel Yugoslavia one evening after one such disappointing event. Dušan was selling his pictures to raise money, but some buyers became irritated when they received copies instead of originals. Dušan, who didn't have enough originals, was humiliated. In my opinion, if they wanted to help, then what difference did it make? I wanted to give all the money we received to his wife, child, and sick mother (who had no source of income), but Dušan went ahead and bought roses, instead, and gave them to all the women present. Dušan, preserving his dignity with a gentlemanly smile, gallantly drove his wheelchair from one table to another, and asked the ladies to take a rose from his lap. But his pride and his desire to act like a gentleman annoyed me because all the money that we had collected ended up in the pocket of a little Roma girl on the street nearby who was selling the roses, which, in turn, ended up in the hands of the ladies who had protested because they didn't get original artwork from a paraplegic who was missing one arm. Fellini may as well have directed this outrageous scene.

The Zemun Municipality had chosen a member of the Radical Party, Vojislav Šešelj, as its President. Rumors about him — that he was a Croat from Herzegovina, were circulating — but most of the world media portrayed him as a Serbian nationalist. He was a Rabelaisian character, at once funny and pathetic. He mythologized himself by issuing controversial statements and engaging in histrionic behavior. These stories left me with an impression of unreliability, but his charisma was attractive. Since I was a member of the Association of Wounded Veterans of this war, and an associate of Good Will, I contacted the authorities in Zemun to see if I could get property to build houses for the Krajina refugees.

Šešelj appointed the President of the Executive Council of the Municipality as his liaison. This fellow was civilized, kind, and helpful. (Later, we learned that he had been murdered under strange circumstances.) He promised to help, provided that several conditions were met. One of these conditions was that I show him the financial plans for the construction of the houses. He told me that he didn't want rumors going around that these disabled vets had sold the property intended for housing in order to squander the money on drink. During this process of obtaining construction plans, I encountered only disappointment, so I became discouraged and pessimistic. None of the Western humanitarian organizations I visited had funds for disabled veterans, and they weren't donating any money or materials for housing construction. So much for humanitarian aid. There were some benefits (reduced apartment rental rates) for those who were employed, but that was all. Much later, we learned that the chief activity of these humanitarian organizations was conducting espionage on behalf of foreign secret service organizations.

The Captain Dragan Fund was also ineffective. I often met with representatives of different so-called humanitarian organizations that were openly struggling for predominance and quarreling in public. The Serbian Orthodox Church was no exception. When I asked for help, I was greeted with the question: *Madam, what do you suppose would happen if all those who needed help lined up in front of the church?* God in heaven, where else are these people going to stand in line for help if not in front of a church? All these meetings ended without finding any significant solutions. I still didn't have any definitive financial plan. But, in the end, the Zemun municipality did donate the property to the disabled vets. My efforts had not been in vain. Šešelj was the only one who kept his word.

I immersed myself in work. I began doing scientific research, to the extent it was possible under the dire economic situation. This did give me a sense of fulfillment. I was completing my doctoral dissertation. I was back in my native Belgrade where I was working at a teaching hospital. I loved my job, but poor working conditions were hampering our effectiveness. We didn't have medicine, and we had no equipment. Harsh sanctions had been imposed on Serbia, so innocent people were dying for lack of medicine and functioning medical equipment. The morgues were full. Patients who had died over the weekend were laying in a long row of stretchers because there was no place to put them. Families didn't even have the money to bury their dead.

Then the war, winding its way among us like a serpent and baring its deadly fangs to whomever dropped his guard, finally arrived in Serbia.

An ambulance brings in a child who was hit by a car. His father is with him. The ambulance brought the father because he has no other means of transportation. He has neither a car nor a telephone, and he doesn't have any money, either. All he has is his child. I feel his desperation when I look into his eyes. I leave the OR to assure him that his boy is going to be fine. He's crying, wiping away tears of joy with his dirty, calloused hands. He turns away so I don't see him. He's ashamed of his poverty. He doesn't have money to buy food. He doesn't even have enough money to return to Stara Pazova, which is where the accident took place. I collect some food from our meager duty rations, which are getting smaller by the day. At least there's enough coffee. I check my wallet for cash, as I did yesterday and the day before. I've lost track of how much money I've handed out to people like this man for bus tickets so that they could get back to their homes or refugee camps.

25. Surprising Changes

My *War Journal* was published in December 1996. At first, I didn't want to publish it, but the fall of Krajina changed my mind. The book was supposed to be published under the title *Between Two Teardrops*, but the publisher retitled it *From Krajina, Which No Longer Exists*. Yes, Krajina is gone. The promotion of the book was organized in conjunction with the annual conference of The Association of Serbian Anesthesiologists and Transfusion Specialists. More than 700 people attended, which exceeded my expectations, but since it was an account of wartime suffering, it wasn't a joyful occasion. History had singled me out to be a chronicler. The serialization of my war journal in *Duga* prompted critics to praise its artistry, which disturbed me. This book wasn't an imaginative exercise. In fact, I wasn't the one who wrote it. Life itself wrote this book. Dostoyevsky once said that no one can write better than life itself.

The book sold quickly, and its profits went to the Good Will Association.

When I presented the book at the Military Center, the auditorium was once again filled to capacity. There were more than 250 people in the audience. You couldn't even get into the Smederevo Library, where the book promotion was held. The event came off resembling a memorial service not only for the war dead but also for Serbia's erstwhile dignity. It was also a requiem for Yugoslavia, the country in which we had been born.

There are frequent demonstrations against Milošević in Belgrade. Students are leading the way. Opposition leaders accompany them. But I'm afraid of crowds, so I stay in the clinic where I'm on duty, and I worry about how many injured and dead we're going to get as a result of these demonstrations.

On March 9, 1991, two young men were killed during a demonstration. Since then, there are fears that more killings could take place. Nevertheless, many of my fellow doctors go out to demonstrate. I'm surprised to find that the children of some of those who hold important positions in political parties (such as JUL (Yugoslav Left) and the SPS (Socialist Party of Serbia)), are on the front lines of the anti-government demonstrations. Entire families — in which the children are pitted against parents — are being torn apart. One colleague, whom I respect, is a hospital director. He's ducking out of work to join the demonstrators. I ask him why he hasn't joined the demonstrators publicly.

His answer is typical: "I have two sons there with their friends. They think they're working for a better, more democratic future. As a parent, I can't help but hope for the best for my children. And yet I'm still concerned for my own wellbeing as well as for my privileged position. I don't have the courage that you have to say what I really think. But my sons gave me an ultimatum: they said they'd be ashamed of me if I didn't join them. And I knew they meant it, so I don't want to alienate them. They mean more to me than my career. So, that's why I went."

The protests are spreading throughout Serbia. They're synchronized so that the demonstrators start banging pots and pans and blowing whistles at the same time in different towns. The symbolic noise is meant to be louder than the propaganda and the lies broadcast by RTS (Radio Television of Serbia) in its daily news programming. Serbia is protesting against its government as well as against the unjust world that's killing it with double standards and sanctions.

Some went to anti-government protests, while the others stayed home to protest the protesters. I'm anxious because I belong to both groups. Are the police going to attack the demonstrators — their own people — again? I tremble at the thought. I would prefer to erase forever from my memory those fearful hours that I spent waiting for the injured to arrive in the Emergency Room. I can't forget it. Fear has crept into my bones.

In Kosovo again — Sheer Hell

By August 1998, Kosovo was in chaos. We weren't being informed by the media of what was really going on there, so we had no way of knowing that a bad situation had just gotten worse. They need help. I volunteer to go with the first group because I don't want young, inexperienced doctors going. My maternal instincts are shielding them.

There's considerable resistance among the hospital staff to volunteering. Nobody wants to go to the front lines, so names are chosen by lot. The KLA (the Albanian "Kosovo Liberation Army") is organizing attacks throughout Kosovo. The police force is on the defensive, so they need doctors and nurses to provide emergency medical care to the wounded. The hospital in Priština has an ethnically mixed medical staff, which means that it can no longer be trusted. JNA forces are conducting their own operations in Kosovo; however, the Army doesn't meddle in police affairs, so this necessitates support from the civilian sector. Thus, the Medical Center was called upon to fill a quota of doctors and nurses. Another anesthesiologist from Priština, a neurosurgeon, an orthopedist, a gastroenterologist, a vascular surgeon, and I go from our hospital. A plastic surgeon from Vojvodina is already there waiting for us. Another group of doctors who are on their way to Peć join us in Kruševac. Our group is staying at The Grand Hotel in Priština's city center. The group going to Peć, where there is growing unrest, is continuing its journey by mini-bus. We wish them luck. We all need luck now.

The media's narrative is that the police force has everything it needs: medicine, equipment, personnel, and all necessary diagnostic tools. But the laboratory in Priština works only until 1:00 p.m. weekdays, and it's closed on weekends. CT (Computed Tomography) scans are available only on weekday mornings, while ultrasound is only available every other day. Suffice it to say that the hospital doesn't even have the capacity to adequately care for multiple trauma cases twenty-four hours a day, which is a minimum requirement. Tensions are running high and rising.

Our team is given a car that barely works. The neurosurgeon drives me from the hotel to the hospital every morning. He's disciplined and responsible. We begin to notice a car — the same car — following us every day. We can't figure out who it is, and, of course, we can't ask anyone because we don't know whom we can trust.

The Press Center is located on the second floor of The Grand Hotel. Every day at 1400 hours, a press conference is held during which a daily report is issued. Journalists from around the world attend to get stories that they will then file with their respective bureaus. None of them ever ventures out to do any independent reporting, but they still seem to get news from places where important events are taking place — which seems strange. How are they getting all these sensational stories that uniformly blame the Serbs for the conflict? These journalists, who never leave the hotel, are writing up news reports as if they were eyewitnesses, and these reports are being broadcast throughout the world.

One day, a press team from Romania tries to go out in the field to a nearby area for a story. They are upset and frightened when they return. They hadn't gotten far before the Albanians threatened them with drawn weapons and forced them to return to the hotel because they said that it wasn't safe to go wandering around the area.

On the other hand, local Serbian journalists aren't relying on the same sources as the foreign journalists. They're reporting that the hospitals are functioning perfectly and that they have the wherewithal to treat police officers wounded in action. In reality, things are quite different. Wounded policemen are taken in downstairs in the Orthopedic Ward. They are crowded into small rooms, packed like sardines. There are flies buzzing around everywhere.

An auxiliary telephone line runs the length of the department. Whenever a new group of wounded policemen arrives, our telephone lines always go dead. It's obviously sabotage by the Albanian staff, but no one questions it. One day, an Albanian nurse shows up with a bomb and threatens to blow the hospital up. We all stood there paralyzed. She's someone we've been working with every day! The bomb fell from her hands and we covered our heads, expecting an explosion, but the bomb didn't go off. It was a dud.

Incidents like this one are exasperating. The conditions under which we're working are unspeakably horrifying. The wounded arrive by ill-equipped police helicopters. They are then offloaded and left to lie like stacks of hay on the floor. They're bringing them in from all over Kosovo. The battles are fierce. Our injured soldiers are so riddled with gunfire that their chances of survival are small. Untrained administrative staff members from the police force were sent into the field to confront the enemy but ended up falling into traps set by mujahedin, who are skilled in guerilla warfare. It's no wonder that they're being brutally killed. Some mujahedin known as the "Gang of Five" lured one such group of green recruits into an ambush where they surrounded them, shot them up, and so riddled them with bullets holes that their bodies might as well have been sieves. Consequently, badly wounded police officers end up occupying all the hospital beds that should be available for other wounded patients. So we have to transfer non-military patients to Belgrade via amateur pilots who use private planes owned by schools and sports teams.

I accompanied the wounded in such ill-equipped police helicopters to Belgrade on several occasions. A wounded patient who was breathing with a portable respirator occupied one whole side of the helicopter. The pilot and I had to shut the door on that side with our feet. Then I had to sit crouched down behind the pilot on the other side. I wasn't going to be able to help the patient during the flight if he suddenly did need help. All I could do was watch him from the corner of my eye. We had to fly at a very low altitude. The Albanians were shooting at us from the ground. In order to avoid the gunfire, the pilot had to fly in a random pattern, veering left, right, up and down. I was always afraid that the helicopter was going to tilt on the side where a patient was lying against the door. The two-hundred-pound patient easily could trip the door open and fall out. I was terrified during the entire trip. After having landed in Belgrade at the VMA helipad, a waiting police officer took me to the Internal Affairs building, where I was going to meet a helicopter pilot to take me back — but the helicopter didn't have enough fuel for the return flight. Besides, the engine was overheated. They hosed down the engine, so it could at least fly to Novi Sad, its home base. It was difficult to understand all this. What happened to the military helicopters, which are much better suited for patient transport? I had already arranged for the patient's admission to the hospital and had submitted the medical report. I sent the patient to the VMA's Emergency Room. They took him instead to the ICU. I was exhausted and furious. I complained to the driver that I had seen real chaos in Kosovo. There was more action taking place in our hospital than on the battlefield. He said nothing. He drove into an underground garage, where he made left and right turns until I didn't have the slightest idea of where we were. I finally understood that I wasn't supposed to know where we were going.

When we finally got into an elevator, the driver remained silent until just before we got out, when he asked me: "Doctor, could you please tell my boss what you just told me?"

"Who's he?" I asked.

"The Chief of the Serbian Police, Mr. Đorđevic and his deputy," he explained.

"Why not? You mean to say they don't know about any of this?"

"They don't, Doctor. Accurate information doesn't always reach the right places. There's a lot of confusion."

"Think they'd believe me?"

"I'd like them to hear it straight from you. They can make up their own minds. At any rate, many of us know you're telling the truth, but it's difficult to make our voices heard."

He led me into an office where a man was sitting bent over a map of Kosovo. The driver introduced me. I was wearing a uniform that was too large for me, so I was unprepared for an introduction. Fortunately, this hunched-over man didn't even bother to look at me; instead, he asked me if I wanted anything to drink. I was thirsty, so I said: Yes, water or some juice. He disappeared and didn't return for a long time. Finally, he came back with a glass of juice.

"I barely managed to find it," he said by way of apology. "We don't have anything here. I can't offer you anything to eat. You must be hungry."

"Thank you. I'm not as hungry as I'm disappointed and angry. I was in Krajina where we transported wounded soldiers via military helicopters — M8s. What are we doing with these sports helicopters? They're completely inadequate — and dangerous for the patients as well as for the crew."

"No one ever told me, Doctor."

"I don't get it. Why hasn't anyone ever explained this to you? Where are the police department's staff doctors? Where's the Army?"

"As far as our staff doctors are concerned, many left the country, just as others have. So we were forced to deal with the situation by recruiting volunteers from civilian institutions. That's why you're here. As far as the Army is concerned, this isn't their war. They're responsible for attacks launched from outside the country, but not for those launched within our borders. That's all there is to it."

We talked for a long time. Our conversation helped assuage my anxieties. He called in two of his colleagues. They listened carefully and gave me advice. We agreed that our team should provide medical assistance only to members of the police force. That was our purpose in Kosovo. Local medical staff would have to be responsible for the others. I was given names, and I was instructed as to how and where to find help if I needed it. I also got information on how to contact the military airport.

After I returned to Priština, I contacted the Army. The next transport was an M8 helicopter. When transporting wounded soldiers, I take a nurse anesthetist with me for training. After bringing the wounded soldiers to the VMA in Belgrade, the helicopter flew to Batajnica for refueling. While the paramedic and I were on board during our return flight, the helicopter began looping without warning. I thought that the pilots must either have been horsing around or that someone was shooting at us again. We were bouncing off the walls! We barely managed to hang on to the rails on the floor to which we locked our legs. When the helicopter finally landed, we were so furious that we wanted to strangle the pilots. Then they apologized. They said that they had simply forgotten that we were on board. Then they told us how difficult their assignment was. The only food they had was canned lunch rations, so they ended up developing hemorrhoids. They didn't even have drinking water, let alone water to take a bath. I couldn't believe it. This didn't fit the picture RTS was presenting, which was that of our soldiers being totally equipped and prepared, possessing all the means and wherewithal to defend the homeland.

So, I ended up transporting patients via helicopter to Belgrade, where a police driver would then drive me back to Priština. Before I arrived at The Grand Hotel on this occasion, the hospital called to say there was an operation that had to be performed. The driver was exhausted after several successive sleepless nights. He didn't have anywhere to sleep except in the car. So, I left him in my hotel room while I went directly to the hospital. I was beyond tired, but the mere mention of an operation got my adrenalin flowing again. A patient whose arm had been severed arrived from Peć. We didn't have time to send him to Belgrade, so we had to try to reattach his arm. We operated on him for more than nine hours in a hospital that didn't even have drinking water. Black, viscous fluid was coming out of the faucets. The temperature outside was 104°F.

The next morning, the patient was able to move his fingers. Those small, tentative movements reinvigorated us. Two days later, I transported him to Belgrade. Later, I learned the police awarded him a medal — but no one mentioned the medical team — the invisible people in white.

During the night, they often brought beardless youths who were doing their compulsory military service. They were dehydrated, scared, and often psychotic. Their eyes were bloodshot and moving wildly, rapidly. They were trembling uncontrollably and they wouldn't let anyone approach them. My colleagues called on me to help. They knew I had some experience with combat-induced psychosis. These young men had been bloodied at the tender age of 18–20. They were given the most difficult assignments a soldier could possibly have received even though they weren't mature enough to endure the horrors of combat.

Their training had been inadequate; their psyches were unable to endure the suffering inflicted on them by their adversaries, the well-trained Kosovo Liberation Army units and mujahedin. In firefights with such opponents, our police officers (many of whom had recently been clerks) and the Army (composed of young conscripts) didn't stand much of a chance. There were cases of suicide among the younger soldiers. The subject was not discussed. We had no choice. This was the only fighting force we had to defend our homeland.

One day, while I was on duty, I went to a kiosk in front of the hospital to buy some juice. After I had gotten the juice and began walking away, an explosion destroyed the kiosk. It was about twenty meters behind me. Even though I was already entering the hospital building, the force of the blast knocked me down anyway. Automatic alarm systems went off in all the cars parked along the street, which created a ghastly spectacle. I barely managed to drag myself into the hospital. I couldn't help but think that the terrorist who blew up the kiosk had waited until I was out of the way. Maybe he wasn't going to wait the next time.

A few days later, I was on duty again at night. Suddenly, a gurney bearing a patient was wheeled into the corridor where it was left between the two units of Intensive Care. We couldn't see him at that distance, so we supposed that he was unconscious. We were wondering who had pushed the gurney in and why no one had accompanied him to inform us of his condition. Maybe he was already dead; maybe the stretcher was full of explosives. We could only guess. The matter had to be resolved immediately, so I took command of the situation. I evacuated the staff and approached the stretcher alone. I wasn't going to let fear control me. An Albanian, as white as a sheet, was lying on the stretcher. His breathing was barely audible. On the left part of his groin lay a small sack with sand. It was an improvised compress. A cannula and a plastic bag with blood were inserted in one arm. I didn't see anything else. We took him to Intensive Care. We gave him oxygen, but we had a problem making an accurate diagnosis because the lab wasn't open. I remembered that we had a centrifuge to test the hematocrit (*i.e.*, the ratio of the volume of red blood cells to the total volume of blood). That would have to do. The results were abnormally low. He was in critical condition. That was why he was so pale. Under the small sack of sand there was evidently an injury to the vein or femoral artery in the groin but I didn't dare remove it. It was terrible.

We had an excellent vascular surgeon who always had an ultrasound device and a microscope with him. I called the surgeons from my team. Until they returned, I went looking for blood but I couldn't find any. Blood is not readily available. I asked the Albanian nurses to help me. They had to find blood for him. They tried but their efforts were unsuccessful. They only managed to find some plasma. I took everything they had.

Now I had the one dose of blood that came with the patient along three 200 ml doses of plasma. The surgeons were already in the OR. I anesthetized him. He was young and he had a strong heart. I asked the Albanian nurses to find his family in order to have them donate blood. He turned out to be one of the leaders of the Kosovo Liberation Army, which was still on the CIA's list of terrorist organizations at the time. He had been wounded in the mountains, where he was treated in a field hospital. When they were no longer able to treat him, they had him brought here through secret channels.

The operation began. His wound was infected. The femoral artery was damaged and inflamed near the groin. The artery was inflamed. He had been bleeding constantly for a long time. The operation lasted the whole night. In the morning, the patient regained consciousness. We didn't have antibiotics and I had no idea where to get some. I again asked the Albanians who worked with us to help. They were afraid. He was from the KLA so they were frightened of retaliation. That didn't make any difference to me. He was our patient. They can arrest him after he recovers, but until then, we had to find antibiotics.

Two days later an Albanian vascular surgeon returned from his vacation. We had already met, so I knew he was a professional. He found antibiotics.

The operation was a success. After a few days, the neurosurgeon took me to the patient's room. Lying in bed, he spoke to us. He told me his name was Ljiljan in understandable Serbian.

"You saved my life. From now on, you're my sister. After our victory, when all this becomes ours, I will give you any house in Priština that you point your finger at."

His words made my flesh crawl. I took his hand and I carefully chose my words: "The most important thing is that you've survived and that you're doing well. Don't worry about the house now. You are the house in which my heart lives."

It was difficult for me to leave him. A conversation with my Albanian friend, Adem B. gave me some comfort. He was tormented by the same feeling. I was overwhelmed with disappointment in my compatriots, while he was disappointed with both Albanians and Serbs. He knew both sides well.

"The Albanians will get Kosovo," he said. "But they will not know what to do with it. Educated secular Albanians have either already left Kosovo or they will be leaving soon. Only the uneducated will remain, and they will be easily manipulated. The Mafia will be everywhere. I feel sorry for Kosovo. This is not the

Kosovo my great-grandfathers dreamed of. This Kosovo isn't going to bring joy to anyone's heart. There's no more happiness here. Joy fled the Balkans long ago. It disappeared along with logical thinking. The Balkan Peninsula is caught between East and West. The different interests of the two worlds have always been in conflict, just as they are today. The nations of the Balkans are just marionettes for any great power that wants to pull their strings. We Muslims didn't need a separate state. No one was threatening us.

"Now our fundamentalists are dragging us backwards two hundred years. The West is taking a leading role in all this, especially the United States. What they need is a disunited Europe. When Europe is on its knees, America beams with pleasure. War in the Balkans means an unstable Europe. Europe is divided as it has always been throughout history. We're going to have a tough time. The U.S. has to transfer its military bases from Germany to Kosovo. We're going to be their servants, cannon fodder for their Army."

* * * *

The Director of Mines in Kosovo, who was also staying at The Grand Hotel, had been the subject of a number of news stories. One day, after I had made his acquaintance, I saw him at the reception desk where we exchanged a few polite words. He left the hotel, and I turned to look for my chauffeur to drive me to the hospital. He was an early riser, so he often had a cup of coffee in the morning and read *Politika* while he was waiting for me. I hardly had time to turn around, when the building was rocked by an explosion. Smoke and flames invaded the hotel lobby. The Director of Mines, who left only a moment before I intended to, had been assassinated. Someone planted a car bomb which was triggered when the driver turned on the ignition. The car was parked right in front of the hotel entrance.

I had to sit down and take a deep breath. My chauffeur appeared immediately. We were so frightened that we didn't dare discuss the incident.

Adem B. didn't come to our meeting at the appointed time. He left me a note at the reception desk advising me that he would meet me in a different location. I was in for a big surprise when we finally did met. He handed me a list of people who had been targeted for assassination. My name was on it. We didn't waste any time asking where it had come from or who had drawn it up. Wasting time trying to answer such questions wasn't going to solve the problem. I had to leave Serbia. I had to flee from whomever it was that drew up the list.

Adem had already made plans for my escape. He chose the new country: Norway. Why Norway? A great number of Albanians had found refuge there, so he knew a lot about the country. He found a place for me where I could learn Norwegian. He downloaded all the information I needed from the Internet. Norway needs 1,000 doctors. He advised me not seek political asylum but to look for work. My brain worked at amazing speed. I devoted all my energy to preparing my escape. I was resolute. From that moment on, there was no room for fear — or mistakes.

On January 16, 1999, the news broke that forty-five Albanians had been killed in Račak. The Serbs were immediately accused of having committed a war crime. The Serbian authorities denied it was a massacre of innocent civilians. They claimed that the deaths occurred during a firefight between the KLA and the Serbian police. The dead Albanians were KLA members. No one believed the Serbian authorities. The International Community was gearing up for its last monstrous operation: the bombardment of Serbia. First, a *pro forma* peace conference was going to be held in Rambouillet where Serbia was going to be offered terms and conditions that no country in the world would have ever accepted. The U.S. negotiated on behalf of the Albanians, so, in effect, Serbian efforts to reach a peaceful agreement had been sabotaged from the start.

26. Operation "Merciful Angel" —
   The Bombardment of Serbia

March 24, 1999 — Smederevo

I'm on my way to an 8:00 p.m. dental appointment. It's been an exhausting day and I'm running a few minutes late. As I'm walking, the sound of a powerful explosion rocks the evening air. It's the first NATO bomb to strike Smederevo.

Immediately after the blast, I hear the wail of air raid sirens. It's a menacing sound that pervades my entire body. My first thought is: *Where are my children?* Then fear and disbelief overwhelm me. I hate NATO. I hate them from the very bottom of my heart. They're bombing my children! I run home as fast as I can. Other people who happen to be caught outside are also running helter-skelter. No one is screaming. We've been struck dumb with fear. We can't believe this is happening to us. How can it be possible that the great 'democratic' world is bombing us and the United Nations is doing nothing to stop it? Isn't there some international law that deals with this? Yes, I'm afraid there is! The law of the jungle: the fittest survive; the weak perish. It has always been so. Democracy is a meaningless word!

I'm out of breath when I reach my apartment, but my girls aren't there. My heart sinks. I don't know where they are. I can't breathe. I ask the neighbors, but no one has seen them. I race back to the center of the town as the sirens continue to wail. A group of frightened people is huddled in front of a building. My daughter Ljuba emerges from the crowd and runs towards me. She's hysterical. She clings to my waist. Her sister Marija is there, too, so both are safe.

"They're going to kill us!" cries Ljuba hysterically. "The bombs are going to kill us. Where are we going to hide?"

Marija is walking around in circles. Then she sits down and started rocking to and fro, moaning indistinctly. I try to gather them in a protective embrace, but their anxiety is so high-pitched that they can't calm down. They're so frightened that I can't even take hold of their hands.

I feel as though I'm suffocating. The children are screaming. I try to calm them down, but it's of no use. We head home to face the uncertain future.

There's no news about the bombardment on TV. Are these mean-spirited traitors, the mass media, going to lie to us again? I'm the only person in our apartment building who has an Internet connection. I find out that the NATO bombardment has begun and that the first bomb has fallen precisely in our vicinity. The bomb struck the military barracks in the village of Vučak, just outside Smederevo. According to the first news reports, no one has been injured.

Neighbors begin coming to our apartment. They're angry, and they're protesting the bombardment. And their questions cut me, too.

"What are you going to do with your children when you go back to work?"

Yes, It's true. I have to report back to work in Belgrade, fifty kilometers away. I have no immediate idea of where I can safely leave my girls.

My neighbors start calming down a little. We begin making practical plans. Dragan and Jelica are going to go to a nearby village, Suvodol. There are no military targets there, so they feel they'll be safer there than here in town. They suggest taking my children with them. I gratefully agree because it solves the problem. But Marija's father then arrives. He too is panic-stricken. We quickly agree that he should take the children, instead. I'm relieved because they aren't going to be with relative strangers. My ex-husband is not an army conscript, so he's able to help. I pack their things for a longer trip, along with a survival kit, too: flashlights, candles, matches. As the world advanced technologically, we're reverting to the candles used by our great-grandparents.

I say good-bye to my girls. I try to stay calm. I don't want them to see how difficult it is for me to part with them. Parting with my children was easier during all the years I spent on the front lines than it is now. At that time, only my life was in danger; now their lives are in danger, too. I feel helpless and unable to protect them.

I return home and try to get some asleep. I'll need every bit of energy I have for what lies ahead. There's no news about either the extent of the bombardment or the resulting injuries. There are no details. The night is eerily quiet. Marko and I talked on the phone three days earlier. He's in Montenegro in rehab after having fractured his leg. He told me that there was tension in the air but that he didn't believe NATO would actually attack us. Bombardment violates all international laws, and it's senseless, anyway, in his opinion. But this nightmare scenario is now unfolding before our very eyes. Being a high-ranking officer, he's expected to return to duty in Belgrade as soon as possible. I wonder whether he'll be able to find a way to get from Montenegro to Belgrade. Many questions remain unanswered. In spite of everything, I have to sleep.

The wars in these regions have lasted for ten years already, so stress has become an inseparable part of everyday life. These ten years have toughened me. I know how to fight, but I also know how to rest. I am as well-disciplined as any soldier. In fact, I *am* a soldier.

I don't know how long I had been asleep when the alarm clock started ringing. I'm lying in bed completely dressed, so I just get up, put on my shoes, take my luggage, and set off for the bus station.

As I leave my building, I'm dazzled by powerful light emanating from the Kovin Bridge, where smoke and flames are belching into the dark sky. The conflagration is lighting up the whole town. A missile hit the Jugopetrol Oil Reserves refinery, which burst into flames. I can't tell if there are any casualties. I also wonder why I didn't hear the explosion. I must have been dead asleep.

My apartment building is dark and silent. The residents have already left town. The parking lot is empty.

The bus station is a five-minute walk away, so I arrive quickly and join a group of people who are already boarding the Belgrade bus. Somehow, we all remain calm. Behind us, flames are engulfing Jugopetrol. Black soot is falling everywhere. We pay for our tickets calmly as if nothing out of the ordinary is happening. We settle into our cold seats as the bus pulls out and gets on the road leading to Belgrade. Ever since the sanctions have been imposed, we've never had enough gasoline. Rumors are circulating that the gasoline shortage is not the result of government rationing but of the authorities allowing drivers to sell black-market gasoline to supplement their meager incomes. There isn't enough gasoline available on the open market, so it's difficult to find a satisfactory explanation.

The bus is so cold that our backsides would have frozen unless we were wearing enough layers of clothing. We have to shift our sitting position frequently. Even inside the bus, caps and gloves are indispensable. I can see my breath. A layer of frost is clinging to my chilblained nose. Many a time since then, I've daydreamed that I had fallen asleep in the cold and had frozen to death with a smile on my face, as did the protagonist in H.C. Andersen's story, *The Little Match Girl.*

It's forty-six kilometers from Smederevo to Belgrade, so the trip usually lasts about forty minutes if the driver takes the highway, or an hour if the driver choses to go by way of Mali Mokri

Lug. I use this hour to rest from all the housework I've done, as well as from the foreboding thoughts that are preoccupying me. Otherwise talkative, I prefer in this situation to remain silent and snooze. I always use the same method: I curl up in a fetal position as I try to stay warm, and I doze off the moment we depart.

Near Bubanj Potok, the bus breaks down. Annoyed, we get off and try to hitch rides with passing cars. This happens all the time because the buses are old and there aren't any spare parts. The sanctions have rolled back twenty years of development. I wonder what new hardships this bombardment has in store for us. Private automobiles are in just as bad a condition as the buses are. But there aren't many cars on the road. We stamp our feet to keep the circulation flowing. Suddenly, the bus engine roars back to life and we gratefully return to our seats. We're frozen stiff.

I get to the medical center on time where I get a message to go to the Emergency Center immediately for a meeting with the department heads. I'm the Head of the Anesthesiology Department for the Otolaryngology Clinic. At the meeting, we're advised that no casualties have been registered after the first night of bombardment. One woman died from a stress-induced heart attack almost in front of the ER, but her life couldn't be saved.

Since I live in Smederevo, I can't commute to work every day. This means that the clinic is going to be my home for an indefinite period of time. Once again, I'm not going to be able to be with my children, but this time they aren't safe. Whenever sirens wail at midnight, and powerful explosions follow, we have no way of knowing the precise location of the strike. Smederevo could be hit but I wouldn't have any way of knowing about it. The bombardment continues until about half past six in the morning when a new siren signals farewell to the deadly planes, which flee at daybreak.

Knez Miloš Street, where the Clinical Center and the School of Medicine are located, is near the Federal Ministry of Internal

Affairs as well as the General Army Headquarters. The Clinical Center consists of a complex of some twenty buildings that house different institutes and hospitals. All the organs of government are in our vicinity. Our patients are not spared powerful blasts that rattle the windows. The constant fear that we might be hit next keeps grinding us down.

We try our best to create an atmosphere of harmony, fellowship, and inner peace. The head nurse picks my brain about my experience in war zones. She then quickly succeeds in creating a work atmosphere similar to the one we had in Krajina. We did manage to overcome our fear of constant danger by having our meals together and by holding daily staff meetings in the same place. We operate casually, and try to remain relaxed. We don't stop living. Disease is still our principal enemy.

At first, we think we should darken the windows but we later give up on the idea. It's impossible to black out the windows in so many buildings, and besides, the enemy doesn't need to see us in order to bomb us. They're firing missiles guided by the target's coordinates. These modern day marauders have precise maps, down to the inch, of Belgrade, a city which the Celts founded in the fourth century B.C. Since then, Belgrade, built at the confluence of the Sava and Danube Rivers, has been bombed by enemies and allies alike thirty-eight times by forty different armies over the centuries. Hitler carpet-bombed Belgrade on April 6, 1941; the Allies carpet-bombed it on Easter Sunday 1944. Belgrade survived those bombardments and it will survive this one, the thirty-ninth.

Serbia is being attacked from all directions. Television screens unleash terrifying images of fire, devastation, charred human remains, and the demolished homes of ordinary people who, if they survive, now have nowhere to go. Psychological warfare is going to cause more harm than the actual material devastation. It's a war of nerves.

A new channel has begun broadcasting from the Parliament Building in Belgrade. It features opposition Members of Parliament, so we're regularly receiving updates from Belgrade, which gives us some reassurance. We feel calmer and we regain a sense of control over our lives. The city has to survive. People can't hide in bomb shelters because we don't have any. The spaces that the city had designated as bomb shelters were long ago converted into cellars and basement apartments. Belgrade has been struggling with serious housing shortages for years. The population of the city has swollen with the arrival of a million refugees since the wars in Krajina, Bosnia, and Kosovo broke out. The panicking population is taking shelter in the few remaining cold, dark, and inhospitable cellars. There are instances of people who took refuge in cellars, where they thought they would be safe. Nevertheless, the missiles that struck these buildings were so devastating that these people were instantly killed. They would have been better off in their apartments. But how can anyone make shrewd decisions and give sound advice at a time like this? Experience is of no use because this new generation of weapons is far more powerful. We're learning that day by day. We learn by seeing the dead and the injured in the smoldering ruins of our country. What hurts the most — more than all the destruction — is the humiliation to which the world has subjected us.

I'm chronically restless. There's no sun in the sky, and there are no stars visible at night. I'm not the only one who's stewing in feverish vulnerability. It's spreading like a contagion and infecting an ever growing number of people. Protests give vent to the anger erupting in the population. In response to this universal tragedy, furious but helpless people are spilling out into the streets. Music begins roaring from loudspeakers in the Trg Republike. Concerts protest the NATO bombardment. The rhythms of music and dancing expend the accumulated adrenalin. The proximity and fellowship of other people creates a sense of unity and strength. At first, there are hundreds of people, then day by day the number of protesters swells rapidly. It's always easier to share. Fear may also be shared, as death may be. They're bombing us, but we stopped worrying. We have more important things to do on Earth. Streets have been painted and are filled with graffiti. Bombs can't stop our creativity. The art created is profoundly existential and genuine. People create in order to survive, to preserve their human dignity in spite of NATO's "merciful bombardment."

Belgrade is the lead singer in the chorus of its own defense. Unarmed and alone in the world, we're singing in reckless disregard of danger. Our resistance allows us to ignore the missiles. They can't bring us to our knees. They can kill us, yes, but they can't defeat us.

* * * *

I was in the hospital, so I couldn't attend the mass demonstrations. Even if I hadn't been busy with patients, I wouldn't have gone. I've always been afraid of crowds. I never go to large concerts or sporting events. I get claustrophobic and I feel as though I'm being suffocated. Even as I was watching television news reports of the masses of people protesting, I was afraid for them. I don't trust NATO.

On April 1, Marko suddenly appeared. He finally managed to find a way to get here from Montenegro. He arrived at my clinic in the afternoon. I loved how he looked in his uniform. We were at a war again! We were in danger again! These were the circumstances under which we had met in Krajina.

I held him tightly.

I hadn't been afraid in Krajina, and I wasn't going to be afraid now. I was, however, afraid for my children, for all the children of Serbia. If they survive, what consequences will the bombardment have on their later development? How are they going to see the world and how are they going to find their place in it? How can justice possibly be achieved by bombardment?

Long columns of small children zigzag through the streets of Belgrade with flowers and flags in their hands. They're singing, and even though their young voices haven't yet cracked, they're showing resistance and they're taking a stand against the invisible pilots. The children are inviting the pilots to come down and play with them, to send them toys and chocolates instead of cruise missiles. These scenes could have been filmed by Sergei Eisenstein. All the details are in place: the spies and the American professionals who are walking around with their notebooks and taking note of Belgraders' reactions to the bombardment. They are treating us as if we were laboratory animals that are being subjected to one of their demonic experiments. Why are they keeping such records? Are they planning to bomb a few other countries too?

April 8, 1999 — Belgrade

Yesterday, I took my first day off since the beginning of the bombardment. I hurried home to Smederevo. I miss my children. The bus line is operating normally but with fewer departures than before. At the bus station in Smederevo, I check on the departure time of the return bus for tomorrow morning. I'm completely unprepared when I walk up to the door of the bus station and I see a death notice posted on the window that knocks the wind out of me. I can't even scream even though I want to scream as loud as I can. It can't possibly be true! His familiar face is smiling at me from the death notice. It's Adem B., my Albanian friend, who worked for the Kosovo police force. He was killed on April 4 in Kosovo. Today — when I just happened to decide to come back to Smederevo — is his funeral. I think of his wife and children. I have to get to the funeral on time. I run stumbling home. Having only an hour before the funeral starts, I'm forced me to pull myself together. I bring yellow flowers wrapped in blue paper, which is customary at Albanian funerals. How cruel and evil life seems. It gnaws at you before suddenly tearing out your heart in one single bite. Why doesn't it just take everything all at once? We'd suffer less that way. Pain has numbed me. Why him? Why should his children be left father-less? How I hate this life.

His wife's words echoed in my mind. She had begged him to return home from Kosovo.

"Come back! Come back!" she insisted. "Leave everything and just come back!"

He hesitated and then said: "I can't! I gave my word to the chief. As long as he's here, I'm going to be here, too."

I supported his decision.

"Let him go and do what has to be done," I said. "You know that he hasn't worked for a long time. He's losing his self-respect. Now he's got this important position. It means a lot to him. It would be unacceptable for him to resign now."

"Why doesn't he just leave everything so we can all go somewhere else?" she asked. "I'm tormented by a sense of fore-boding, a premonition of evil. I don't know how to express it in words."

"Why don't you study for your exam while I'm gone?" Adem advised her. "You could pass your neuro-psychiatry board exam. Make the most of your time while I'm away."

My head is spinning. Thoughts come fast, tumbling over each other.

My lips tremble as I remember one August day in 1998 in Priština when I was working there as a doctor. Adem was work-ing as an advisor to the director of the local MUP office there. I often felt desperate. Strange things were happening. Humanitari-an organizations were setting up shop in Priština. I recognized many of their representatives from previous contacts in Belgrade through the Association of Disabled Veterans. None of them ever contributed a penny to the disabled, and they had even ridiculed me. They were simply spying on us. I was surprised when I recognized a German man from a well-known humanitarian organization, whose business card I had even received, who was disguised as a nun at The Grand Hotel. Nothing surprised me anymore. They were all criminals. I confided in Adem about what I'd seen. He acted quickly and, after a short conversation with the police, he came back. We found him in the lobby. Adem told me to go into the elevator where the German disguised as a nun was standing. I "accidentally" pressed the button that stopped the elevator. Then the door opened. The police came into the elevator and escorted the German out. The "nun" took off her wimple, and revealed herself to be the man I had recognized. He was wearing combat boots under his nun's habit. I was ill at ease for a long time after this incident. What are these people doing here? Who are they? The more I saw, the more I came to assume I didn't have long to live because death was shadowing us. My late husband had seen too much, so he knew too much. He and others like him were slowly disappearing. Adem had warned me that I too had seen too much. He was gone now, so I was wondering when it was going to be my turn.

All those memories of our conversations in Kosovo in 1998 accompanied me to the cemetery, where a great many mourners had already assembled. His director was, of course, present. We looked at each other over his coffin. My blood ran cold when I saw him. Adem had spoken of him many times. He told me about his positive traits as well as his professional incompetence. He was serving up a lawyerly defense of his boss. There was no need for Adem to defend him, as far as I was concerned. I had never been against the man. But Adem felt compelled to explain the gravity of his position. Perhaps that was how he was trying to explain his own difficult position, one that ended up costing him his life. This is a dirty war. You can't keep your hands clean no matter how hard you try. When you are constantly being forced to maneuver between visible and invisible interests, you inevitably step into a hidden mine field. There is always someone who doesn't like you. Being the head of the MUP Office in Priština is a tough job, but no one ever trusted him anyway.

After the funeral, Adi's wife told me how he was killed — or, shall we say, what she was told about the way he died. I found it strange that Adi had called his wife only a few minutes before he died and that he had told her that he loved her. Did he know that he was going to be killed? How could he have known that a grenade was going to explode in the Post Office — where he just happened to be? Questions that I thought were better not to ask began plaguing me. I still had unanswered questions about my husband's death. I was living in a mysterious nightmare where fear predominated. I was dying slowly. Nothing scares the dead, nor can anything frighten those of us who are the walking dead.

Everyone at work takes note of my grief. Their faces cloud over after I tell them about what happened. They then understand what I'm going through. It doesn't help the atmosphere at work. I'm going to have to control my emotions. As we pass our days living under bombardment, the people around me seem to draw strength from reservoirs they didn't know they had. Our sense of humor returns. We call the sirens before the air raid *šizele* (go crazy), and the ones signaling the end of the bombardment were called *klara* (be calm). We joke about the situation. We just can't let ourselves feel like jack rabbits that NATO bombers are chasing down an open field. Between bombing raids, I give some thought to the Americans' motives for interfering in our country's affairs, for appointing themselves as sole arbiters, and for imposing their will on others by force. How long is this going to last? I wonder.

April 9, 1999

My Aunt Jelena, my father's only sister, was killed. I wasn't even able to attend her funeral. She was found bent over a fence in front of her house. She had been watching NATO aircraft flying overhead. The train that my family was supposed to take to attend her funeral was bombed on the bridge over the Grdelička Gorge. Fifty-two people were killed, dismembered, blown to bits. The pilot was probably hee-hawing at his success in destroying the bridge, the train, and killing so many people in one fell swoop. All we had to be happy about was that my mother and brother hadn't taken that train. Random horror and death are an everyday occurrence.

April 14, 1999

Today NATO bombed a column of Albanian refugees. About a hundred old men, women, and children were killed. It was dreadful! A picture of a crying boy who was wearing a yellow sweater was broadcast on all our TV news programs. A pilot had simply spotted a convoy of tractors just as another had spotted a train going over the bridge at the Grdelička Gorge. NATO deliberately bombed these poor people. There's no other explanation. Did they think that the tractors belonged to Serbs, just as they had supposed the train was Serbian? Who knows? All of us saw the televised images of NATO planes descending for a bombing run over Korisa. Children are losing their lives: a weeping Albanian boy in Belgrade; a wounded Croatian girl or a Serbian boy blown up by a cluster bomb in Krajina; a lost child in Bosnia. It's heartbreaking. Only God knows what dreadful disabilities they will end up with. I don't even know what I'll think about all this tomorrow. I don't know whether I'll think differently tomorrow. I just don't know. I'm filled with hatred and despair.

April 20, 1999

I'm exhausted by stress, I'm frightened, and I'm helpless. We can't protect our loved ones. It's disheartening and depressing, but we're lucky to be working. Work is the best therapy. You focus on the task at hand instead of on things that no one can do anything about. That was how we survived in Krajina when we were working in total isolation. Now, that same feeling of hopelessness is recurring here. The subject of my doctoral thesis was stress. Now I give lectures on how to recognize the symptoms of stress, how to control it, and how to accept the fact that we have every right to be frightened. This is how I begin my lectures: "I'm addressing you, the descendants of those who survived the Balkan Wars as well as the First and Second World Wars. You will survive this war just as your ancestors did the others. We have gathered here today to learn how to survive."

NATO is celebrating its fiftieth anniversary. It is older than I am but I don't even know why it had to be created. At this moment, NATO is an evil, vain, and unmanageable monster. All the bridges in Novi Sad have been bombed. The Bridge of Liberty was blown up in the name of fairness. Whose justice is that? Today, NATO destroyed transformer stations in the Belgrade suburbs. In downtown Belgrade, *TV Bastille* went up in flames. (We call RTS, the state television broadcaster, *TV Bastille* because most everyone disagrees with their politics.) About twenty people were killed, but no journalists were among the victims. News personnel had escaped the effects of the bombardment up to now. Tons of rubble and masonry came crashing down on innocent employees in the broadcast studios. One unfortunate man's leg was jammed between two blocks of concrete. He was dangling upside down, swaying, dead. The medical team from the Emergency Center came to get him down. A crane took them up to the second floor, where they had to amputate the poor man's legs in order to lower his body to the ground.

I am pushing the limits of exhaustion. The nights are dismal. The days begin with a siren announcing the beginning of the bombardment, and they end just before dawn with a siren signaling the end of bombardment. This is the thirty-first day of bombardment.

Still April 1999

I can't think or write any more. My pen moves across the blank page only with difficulty. We perform operations, but we have trouble procuring medicine and equipment. There are no antibiotics, there are no cannulas, and there are no muscle relaxants. A journalist from the *Frankfurt News* called to tell me that a Serbian woman in Vienna wants to send us some of the supplies we need. I get in touch with her and I ask her to send cannulas for children. The whole city of Belgrade needs cannulas for children. If I manage to get them, I can trade them at the Institute for Mother and Child for muscle relaxants. I've become a dealer. I wheel and deal. Somehow, we manage to keep the clinic going.

The authorities have complicated the issue of humanitarian aid. They don't want humanitarian aid to be earmarked for any specific purpose. They want all donations to be stockpiled in one location for later distribution. We're all suspicious of this policy. Humanitarian aid often ended up on the shelves of private pharmacies. Potential donors, having already been made aware of this, are now less willing to lend support unless they know the identity of the recipients. They want to help, but they will more readily send aid directly to people they know, thereby guaranteeing that their contributions of medicine and medical supplies won't end up on the black market. I spend hours and hours on the telephone with these contacts, assuring them that the aid is going to be delivered directly to me — in my name as the official recipient — at the Otorhinolaryngology Clinic.

The woman from Vienna doesn't want to send her aid to the central clearing house. She wants to be sure it's going to benefit our patients directly. I promise to do everything I can. In the end, a shipment of several thousand cannulas for children arrives and, after numerous problems — including disputes with customs officials — do I manage to bring the shipment to our clinic. Then I start wheeling and dealing. I send these cannulas to both children's hospitals in the city, and in return I get larger cannulas for adults or something else they have but that we don't.

May 1, 1999 — Belgrade

I woke up this morning in a hospital bed. Last night, I went to bed at about midnight after an emergency biopsy of an esophagus. It had been more than forty-eight hours since I last slept. Oppressed by fear and fatigue, I heard the sounds of our PVO Air Defense system. The linden tree murmured in protest beneath the window of the room where I slept. I was so tired that I thought I was hearing the sound of the falling rain. Lightning flashed through my closed eyelids. I was expecting my bed to start shaking and the glass in the windows panes to start rattling. I have to get back to work because another bomb has fallen somewhere near the hospital, destroying yet another government building. Day by day, NATO is demolishing Belgrade. It's painful to watch.

Even as I'm writing this, rampant images are running uncontrollably through my conscious mind. They're flashbacks and they're coming one after the other, over and over again. I can't breathe. Flashbacks of destruction jostle against each other, stampede to get out of my mind as fast as they can but my hand can't write as fast as they're stampeding.

I'm reassured by the birds chirping in the bright morning air. I don't dare move. I'm afraid that someone is going to tell me that the last of Belgrade's bridges has been blown up during the night. I'm attached to the Pančevo Bridge. It stretches across the Danube and connects Vojvodina to old Belgrade. Over there, on the other side of the river, my late father lies buried in a beautiful plain. He spent his whole working life draining swampland which he turned into fertile fields where PKB (an industrial farm and food processing concern headquartered in Belgrade) cultivated grain, corn, sunflowers, and many other industrial plants. He loved those green and yellow fields. That's where he wanted to be buried. If that bridge were to be destroyed, then I wouldn't be able to visit his grave. Hundreds of thousands of people would be cut off from their workplaces on the other side of the Danube. On the other side is the Branko Bridge over the Sava River, which leads to Zemun, where I was born. Belgrade needs both bridges to function normally.

Marko was on duty yesterday. That means that we'll be able to see each another after he reports to General Vukadinović, the Commander in charge of the defense of Belgrade. Marko received a promotion during these six weeks since the bombing started. This war helped him once again become the good old officer he used to be. He had begun losing confidence in himself, as well as his self-respect, since he arrived from Krajina in August 1995. The Yugoslav Army High Command was responsible for his falling spirits. They favored people who had been in Belgrade; meanwhile, they heaped scorn on those who had spent five years fighting in Krajina. That hurt the most. He had lost everything: his apartment as well as that part of his family that chose to remain in Slovenia after it seceded from Yugoslavia. He also lost his new home in Krajina. It remained in Croatia, as did his home town, Benkovac. He had nothing. What hurt the most was that the Army, to which he had pledged allegiance, was now stripping him of his dignity. It was sad to watch him grow old before my eyes. He seemed to be getting smaller and more wrinkled.

The loss of identity is the most serious disorder a person can suffer. I fell in love with Marko when he was a capable and decisive officer, a patriot, and an honorable man among many who were not. And now these years of helplessness were killing him. It was hard to watch. For a long time, he didn't have a job or an apartment. He lived with me in Smederevo. It was hard on him. Disappointed and angry, I wrote to General Perišić, the Commander of the Yugoslav Army at that time, about Marko's situation. I didn't think anything would come of it. But it resulted in Marko being called in for an interview, after which he was assigned to a new post. Then he lost that job, as well. Marko suffered a stroke, then later he broke his leg. When the bombing raids started, he was in a rehabilitation program in Montenegro where he was recuperating from the broken leg.

Now, a few weeks into the bombing campaign, Marko once again became that old commander I knew from Glina and Knin. He functions best in wartime. Danger is his natural milieu. It reinvigorated him and he became more cheerful. His skin became taut again. He's active. In only two weeks, he was promoted to second in command to Gen. Vukadinović. Marko is responsible for all technical matters. He organizes the demolition of ruins and the clearing of rubble. He's also in charge of sequestering damaged structures and of protecting inhabitants from any possible building collapse. He's responsible for the water distribution system, the electrical grid, sewage system, and a host of other things.

So, the opportunity for us to meet never presents itself even though we live only a few kilometers apart. Even when we speak on the phone, we have to resort to official discourse. We're at war and I'm in love with a high-ranking officer who has burdensome responsibilities. I learned the unspoken rules of conduct when we were in Krajina. That's why I'm happy to see him whenever I can. When we're both off duty, we can organize our time fairly well. Then we go to Sarajevska 9 where Marko has a

300 square-foot studio apartment. That's the only place where the two of us can be alone for a short while. We miss our privacy. I'm at the hospital all the time, up all night, and walking the razor's edge all day long. As Department Head, I have my hands full trying to keep things functioning normally with less resources — financial and otherwise — than necessary, although we do have some reserves in case of mass injuries. Patients come to the hospital, we perform the operation, and then we send them home. The scope of our effectiveness is reduced, but at least the department is functioning.

At night, we often take in choking cases, so we frequently operate on the throat and windpipe. People are nervous, and they aren't chewing and swallowing their food properly, so bits of food get trapped in the windpipe instead of going down the gullet. They often bring children. Parents are tense and they're being ground down further with each passing day, so they're less capable of caring for their children than they were before. We can hear the planes buzzing overhead, and they're keeping us awake and on guard all night long.

Tonight, for the second time since the NATO bombardment began, I'm leaving the clinic to be alone with Marko. I'm the only anesthesiologist on duty in the hospital. I got into habits that I couldn't have changed even if I had wanted to. By staying up together night after night at the hospital, we members of the staff created new relationships. Danger had brought us together. Tonight, I had to ask a doctor to replace me on duty. She was already there, ready and waiting, but the rest of the staff protested because I was leaving the clinic. They feel safer when I'm with them.

Something tragic happened last night. We were sitting down to our usual meal together after having made the evening rounds in the ward. Nurses who traveled to work from distant parts of the city were telling us how different people were coping with the bombardment. Besides tragic details, there were also comic ones, so we could enjoy a few laughs. We were happy that NATO was bombing paper and balsa wood decoy planes that the Army had positioned on the tarmac at the military airport in Batajnica. They had devastating weapons which they were using imprudently, but all we had left was clever artifice and a good laugh.

As we were talking, a dark shadow swept past the window. Someone asked:

"What was that? Those gravediggers (*i.e.*, NATO) must have started firing soundless missiles. They already have invisible planes. Who knows what else they're going to throw at us!"

We all laughed, but suddenly an unpleasant thought crossed my mind. I ran outside to check whether my forebodings were justified. The others followed me. We all came to the same conclusion at the same time. Unfortunately, we were right. In front of the hospital lay the body of one of our patients in an unnaturally twisted position. It was a suicide, one more in a long series that began with the bombardment. It's especially hard for our patients who've had operations for throat cancer. They can't speak, they can't eat, and they suffer severe pain. We're not able to help them much. We don't have pain killers. Ever since the sanctions have been imposed, there are shortages of almost everything, especially anesthetics. These patients were now doomed to suffer terrible pain. The number of suicides is increasing daily. Patients jump from the roof of the hospital. A fall from the fifth floor means certain death. None have survived so far.

I ran downstairs and knelt before this patient. His head was twisted abnormally. His neck was broken. A green liquid — gastric juices from his empty stomach — was running from his mouth. He was hungry when he died.

The sanctions are leaving their deadly mark on all aspects of our lives. Its vivid effects can be seen on our patients. It was a relief to finally leave the Emergency Medical Center. I accepted a new position as the Department Head of Anesthesia at the Otorhinolaryngology Hospital because I could no longer stand to see so many of our patients dying. We could have healed them if we had only had the necessary medicines and functioning medical equipment. From time to time, we run out of intravenous nutritional infusions. There are days when we have only two half-liter bottles of saline solution for eighteen patients, each of whom needs at least three liters to sustain vital functions. They're all on respirators so there's no chance of them eating normally. Our respirators frequently break down. Here in the Otorhinolaryngology Hospital, the situation is similar to the Emergency Medical Center. The only difference is that patients are dying quickly in the Emergency Medical Center due to untreated illnesses or injuries that cause unmanageable complications, while here they are dying slowly because we don't have medicine. In the past, we could have treated them successfully. There's no escape from the consequences of impoverishment.

27. Coping with Every Day Misery

Marko's son, Vladimir, and the son of General Pavković, the Commander of the Yugoslav Army who is now stationed in Kosovo, share Marko's tiny apartment on Sarajevska Street. Vladimir is a friend of the General's son from his first marriage. He and his mother came from Čapljina in Bosnia, where they had suffered a long imprisonment in Dertelj, a Muslim prisoner-of-war camp. They then lived in a small room in a military annex in Zvezdara. Other officers who had been banished from territories of the former Yugoslavia were living in cramped lodgings, where four-to-six people shared a room stacked with bunk beds. So, the young man would often come to Sarajevska Street where there was more room. Marko and I could sleep at work in order to give the boys more living space. The apartment is modestly furnished. There's no telephone because we don't have enough money to have one installed. Nor do we have the money to buy a cell phone. The Army is unable to provide Marko with one. That's just the way it is. This guy takes care of two million people in Belgrade, but he doesn't have a cell phone to coordinate with the Red Cross and other organizations. This war is corrupting everything, so it's no wonder that we're losing it. If the unjust world had been our only enemy, it might have been easier. But we were fighting two wars, one against the unjust world, and the other against the political mafia. We're all short of money and we're getting poorer by the day. Whenever the Army couldn't help, we relied on friends and their connections. A fellow doctor's brother wanted to help the Army in a symbolic way, so he gave Marko a mobile phone and installed a landline in his apartment. That's life under the sanctions.

Marko arrives on time for our long anticipated rendezvous. He brings cigarettes for my staff. He's not a smoker, but he regularly takes the Army's cigarette rations and hands them out to his friends. I also have a reserve stash of cigarettes in my cupboard that I can give to friends if they start getting jittery. They sometimes sell cigarettes in a kiosk by the hospital, where people stand in long lines to get them. Although I did not smoke, I sometimes waited in line to buy a pack or two to have on hand for nerve-wracked people who needed a smoke. Once, while I was standing in line, I had to laugh at a sticker on the kiosk that read: *We are the only country in the world where people stand in line to get cancer from smoking.*

Once again, it's a comic take on an impossible situation.

Branko is on duty for the night shift, so he and Goran the anesthetist get the cigarettes directly from Marko. They wave as we drive away in our green Yugoslav-Army-issue Opel to Marko's cozy little apartment. I carry plastic bags of food, towels, and toilet paper. Onions, lettuce, red radishes, and warm rolls are coming right up. Spring came a while ago, but we haven't yet had the chance to enjoy the fruits of the earth. Marko has all his gear, too. The apartment is tidy. The boys have gone to spend the night at the military annex. That's not how we'd have liked it to be, but it's the only way we can get some privacy. Marko and I have, after all, the right to spend a few hours together. It's our right to give effect to the most basic of human needs. Love and tenderness give us strength and shield us from insanity. A person who is in love isn't going to hurt or kill someone else.

We don't have much time. We know that death may easily part us at any moment, so we're attentive to each other. This is the only time I feel safe, secure, and protected. I talk and talk, making all sorts of vows and promises. I'm happy simply because we're together. But my Colonel is the silent type. Nary a word from his lips — only kisses. That's what he's like. I'm the talkative one. Marko falls asleep on my breast. I love caressing him with my eyes, watching over him as he sleeps. I'm careful not to awaken him.

We're alone together for the first time since the bombardment has begun. Marko's Motorola cell phone is his only connection with headquarters. He has to leave it on. Voices begin crackling in the darkness:

> Zlatibor calling Bor ... there's a plane at elevation 6. It's going towards Branko's Bridge!

> Peručica calling Maljena ... rocket at elevation 3! Take action! Zivota please respond? What happened Života?

> Nothing! Fuck it!

This goes on for a whole hour. During the night, planes and missiles are coming from the north as well as the south and they're all heading for Belgrade. The PVO Air Defense is returning fire. A very skillful Života, if that's his real name, takes down a missile above Branko's Bridge. Our anti-aircraft fire forces two NATO planes above the bridge to change direction. Later, one of the planes drops its payload on a less important target. The CK Building (Central Committee of the Communist Party of Yugoslavia), located in the Ušće neighborhood at the confluence of the two rivers, is on fire. We hear the explosion, then a violent blast of air flings open the windows of our room. Marko jumps up and gets dressed in the dark in the matter of seconds.

> *Eagle calling* Falcon*! Can you read?*
> *Tsvrrrr ... krrrrr ... krrrr....*

And then nothing. The cell phone stops working.

Marko arranged to have a driver meet him on the street in front of the apartment should a missile strike, so he's not particularly upset about the cell phone. A deal is a deal, and the driver will be here if he's still alive. Marko is annoyed by the loud music coming from a nearby bar. It always makes him angry that there are people who behave in an undignified manner during the bombardment. For some, it's a real war; for others, however, it's an excuse to party. If people were as good as Marko had wanted them to be, then there wouldn't be any wars at all.

Once we hear the sound of the car engine outside, Marko bounds down the stairs and out the door.

I stand at the window fully dressed and wave to the car as it pulls away. Then I lie down fully dressed again on the empty bed. I began shivering with anxiety, helplessness, and despair. Even if something should happen to him, I doubt that anyone will be in a hurry to notify me.

I love him.

I have to remain silent. It's harder for him than for me. The Avala TV Tower has been destroyed. It was the symbol of Belgrade, just as the Eiffel Tower is to Paris and the Statue of Liberty to New York City. The Avala Tower was built in 1965, and it stood prominently in view from no matter what direction you approached Belgrade. It rose above the city like a guardian. On many occasions, my heart warmed at the first sight of that Tower in the distance as I was returning home from a trip. It imparted a feeling of security. Just one single NATO cruise missile made it disappear. Another explosion destroyed the radio transmitter in Krnjača. I'll never forgive them.

I'm unhappy and desperate on my way back to the hospital. I want to scream. I have to do something. In my anger and misery, I told Marko that I wanted to be mobilized to fight if NATO begins a land invasion. I wasn't going to let those villains kill my children. I'd shield them with my own body. We were passing the Ministry of Foreign Affairs building, where the magnificent crest of the magnolia tree was glowing under the streetlights. What would happen if this building were to be blown up? We'd build a new one in a few years, but it would take more than twenty years for a magnolia to grow to such a height and blossom with such large flowers as it has tonight. This bombardment is irreversibly upsetting the balance of nature. Besides killing people, it's destroying vegetation, contaminating the air and soil, and polluting all the rest. Nature is never going to forgive them. Tulips of many different colors, which are planted in front of the building, scent the nighttime air. I love tulips. This spring their scent is particularly intense. Extraordinary fragrances fill the earth. Nature seems more pronounced than before. The greenness of the grass has never been so intense, while the dandelions resemble small, yellow suns. Now I feel a dull pain in my heart. I'm afraid for all this beauty.

As I'm heading toward the Otorhinolaryngology Hospital (and carrying my dirty laundry in a plastic bag), my high-heels beat a regular rhythm on the asphalt. I planned to hand-wash my laundry at the hospital, but nothing is going according to plan. I ring the bell, then the night watchman opens the door. He's drunk, and he has a bandage on his forehead, which makes me wonder what he's been up to. Lately, he's been depressed. But alcohol isn't going to make him forget the war or make him deaf to the sound of exploding cruise missiles. I say *Good evening* to him, but he doesn't even hear me. I take my laundry to the second floor, and leave the night watchman to nurse his hangover. A colleague is sleeping in the apartment reserved for the on-duty anesthesiologist on the third floor. This apartment has been set aside for special patients and important politicians. Since I have nowhere else to go, the Director lets me use it. It have a private bathroom, which means a great deal to me. I can relax. I escape the scrutiny of those who are looking for signs of fear in my face. I enter the room quietly and see that my colleague is awake.

"What happened? What did they bomb now?"

"Avala! Krnjača! Marko had to go," I say.

"O, my God! Avala … Avala! They really *are* criminals. Did Marko have to go there?"

"Yes. I'm afraid for him."

"Be optimistic. Try to think about something else. You've always been positive and you've encouraged us. Don't you lose courage now."

We go to bed. I try to fall asleep. Soon, I have an oppressive nightmare that drags me into an abyss of hyperexhaustion.

Fijuuuuuuu! Gruuuuuuuummmm! is the sound a cruise missile makes. We can hear them roaring all night long.

The windows of our room are flung open by a violent blast that knocks my colleague right out of bed. The next moment, we both get up on our feet, get dressed, and run out into the corridor to check up on our patients. Many are already bewildered, running to the stairs, their faces contorted by grimaces of fear, helplessness, and horror. I yank the gown of the first patient I reach, who is panting through his cannula and is unable to say anything. His feeding tube is wrapped around his head, so in the semidarkness he looks more like a sci-fi creature. He can't speak because his vocal cords have been cut. Since he can't scream, his eyes are bugging out. The inability to verbally express horror is particularly difficult. When the bombardment first began, the patients used to run out into the corridor where they would vomit. That was the only way we could hear them. We're just as frightened as they are, but we have to calm them down. I put my hand on one patient's chest. His heart is pounding wildly, as if it wants to leap out of his rib cage. This particular heart is suffering too much stress: operations, X-ray treatment, lack of medications, hunger. He just couldn't take the bombing any longer. There are no *humane* reasons to kill the sick and wounded, as NATO is now doing.

Patients are advancing toward me from every direction and they're pushing me toward the stairs. I lose my balance from the onslaught and fall hard onto the concrete floor. Luckily, my head lands on someone's hand, which breaks my fall. I feel the stampeding patients trampling me, so I shield my head with my arms. After a minute or two, the patients start calming down. Someone gives me a hand to help me up. I can barely stand on my left foot. My hip and shoulder are bruised and they hurt like hell, but it could have been much worse. I immediately turn my attention to the patients. I'm especially concerned about the ones who are confused and staring at me. I ask them in the most soothing voice I can summon, all the while assuring them that everything is going to be all right, to return to their rooms. It's not the first time that NATO has bombed a target so close to the clinic. We all have to exercise self-control. After the patients are all safely back in their rooms, the staff climbs to the roof of the clinic, which is off limits — but we go there anyway. There, we have a panoramic view of the city. There's a beautiful full moon above. Looking north, the Medical Center building blocks our view, so we can only see the rising smoke. Did they bomb the MUP near the Gazelle Bridge? We see flames and smoke toward the south, coming from the direction of the Beogradjanka Palace.

We wonder aloud whether the Pančevo Bridge or the Army Headquarters has been bombed. A moment later, we're certain that Army Headquarters has been hit. It's just as I had supposed. Another strong sudden blast hits us from behind. The lime tree in front of the hospital — that one that once stood as high as the roof — has been uprooted and has vanished into the darkness below. Leaves flutter in the air. I turn instinctively in the direction of the sound just in time to see two red balls of fire coming towards us. I can't estimate the distance, the height or the size, but they're unstoppable. It seems that they're coming right at us. A surgeon was standing in front of me is talking on his cell phone. He doesn't see the approaching fireball. There's no time to say anything. I yank his sleeve and we both fall into the corridor of Department C. Another strong explosion sends a sweeping blast of air through the open door that is so powerful it slams us up against the wall. We don't know what hit us. We get up, and in a heartbeat were back on the roof again.

A black mushroom cloud rises from the direction of Army Headquarters. Whorls of smoke rise from the lower floors as sharp, yellow flames lick the sides of the building. O, my God, is this an atomic bomb?! The scene resembles Hiroshima. I can't believe it. I'm paralyzed by shock, but another more distressing thought flashes through my mind. I know Marko is near the Army Headquarters. I saw his green Opel accelerate down the street behind the hospital towards the burning building. Only 200 meters in a straight line separate us. When the second cruise missile hit Army Headquarters, he was surely there. If that's true, then he may be injured or even dead.

"Nooo!" I scream uncontrollably.

My colleagues know why I'm screaming. Someone embraces me and starts talking to me. I hear nothing, absolutely nothing. I can't stop thinking about him. I'm having convulsions. I lose my voice. Another thought flashes through my mind: *If he's hurt, he's going be brought to the Medical Center.* This is the nearest hospital. I bolt down the stairs two at a time. I run out into the street and make straight for Army Headquarters. I'm wearing only my short-sleeved uniform and hospital clogs. I'm not wearing any stockings, but I don't feel the cold at all.

Down by the access bridge to the Medical Center, a red fire engine stops in the middle of the street. The windshield is shattered. The passenger-side windows don't have a single pane of glass. The engine body is riddled with bullet holes. The cab door opens right in front of me and I step right into a pool of blood pouring from the leg of an injured man. His leg is dangling unnaturally. The firemen who bring him ask me to help. I take the pale bulky man by one arm, while a fireman from inside the cab holds the other. We place him on a stretcher and wheel him into the Center. We find out he's a member of the city council and that he was injured right in front of the Ministry of Foreign Affairs. But I don't have time to listen to his story.

"Are there any more?" I ask the firemen anxiously.

"Plenty! A lot of 'em are still in the street!" shouts the fireman leading the team.

"I'm going with you!" I say quickly. "Just let me get my first aid kit."

I run into the Medical Center. Someone grabs me by my uniform and says: "Are you crazy? You'll get yourself killed!"

I tear myself away. The nurses in the Casualty Ward give me a first aid kit, but they also urge me to stay with them instead. No, I can't do that. Not tonight. I run toward the departing fire engine and I almost get hit by a car that's going the wrong way down the street. It's a Russian Lada bringing in another victim. The driver is frightened and exhausted. I see a bearded man lying in the back seat who looks so pale that he may not have had a single drop of blood left. His legs have been traumatically amputated below the knees, crushed and slung over what remains of his thighs. It sends a chill down my spine.

"Help! He's bleeding heavily," I shout to the crowd moving about. "Quick!"

Now I'm shouting at someone who's walking toward me: "Get the gurney over here right now! We need an oxygen mask!"

A team of doctors arrives instantly and we quickly get the man on a gurney. The fire engine in the distance honks its horn. I leave everything and I jump into the back seat. The fire engine drives through the darkness of Knez Miloš Street. My feet are in a pool of blood on the floor. It's hell.

On the street near the Ministry, we see heaps of rubble, broken pieces of asphalt, and tangled iron work. The fire truck jostles as it navigates pot holes. There's an undamaged luxury vehicle parked on the asphalt. On the left, at the traffic light, there's a metallic gray BMW. It also looks undamaged. On the right are trees whose trunks have been broken in half. The twisted wreck of a mushroom-shaped bus stop shelter has been ripped from its foundation. It's a grotesque scene. The firemen tell us that members of the Belgrade municipal government have been killed. They left their car after the first cruise missile struck, only to be hit by the second. For the first time since the bombardment began, the same place has been bombed twice. Anyone who happened to be coming to the rescue was killed. A silent scream is trapped in my throat.

I avert my eyes from the demolished building only with difficulty. In the dusty and smoky semi-obscurity, I discern some dim lights two-to-three hundred meters away. Beyond that, I can see the movement of vehicles and people. I look for Army Headquarters on the right, a little further up. It just might end up being Marko's tomb. As we make our way across the rubble-strewn intersection, I ask the firemen if there are Army casualties. Yes, they say. Four, either dead or wounded.

"Where are they now?" I ask, pressing the question.

"A military ambulance picked them up. There aren't enough civilian ambulances in good working order."

They show me the spot where the guard post used to be. All that's left is a crater in the asphalt. Nothing's left. When we cross the intersection, I see the building housing the Serbian Seat of Government. Its doors and windows have been blasted out. This used to be a grand old building. Some of the buildings in Belgrade predate the founding of the United States. The sanctions are destroying us, and the bombardment is destroying whatever the sanctions didn't.

My attention is drawn to the flames rising high behind Army Headquarters, where two silhouettes are moving through a passageway between buildings. They're coming towards us. One moment the fire is smoldering and calm; then the next it flares, shoots up high, and lights up the entire area. In one such burst, I recognize the shadows approaching us.

"Marko!" I shout, completely out of control.

The firemen look at me in surprise.

"I'm sorry!" I say, apologizing. "That's my man over there. I've been looking for him."

They immediately stop the fire engine. I open the door of the cab and ran towards Marko. The street is wide but strewn with rubble. I feel as though I'm flying. Marko recognizes me, and starts crossing the street in my direction. In a moment, we're in each other's arms.

He embraces me protectively but then asks me in an official tone of voice: "Do you know how many casualties the Medical Center took in?"

"I know of two," I reply. "I went with the firemen when they asked me to help. We didn't see anyone who was injured along the way."

"Go back with them. I have to cordon off the area."

I'm not ready to let him go.

"Just one more second," I say, clutching him. "Where's your escort?"

"Injured," he says, looking at me gravely. "I was only a few meters away when they were hit. It's not the first time I had a close call."

The second shadow catches up with us.

"Bad idea for civilians to be out here," he says.

"She's not a civilian, Comrade General. This is Doctor Sarah," says Marko quietly.

"She out of her mind or what?" asks the General, the one in command of the defense of Belgrade.

Marko keeps his cool but he's holding me so tightly that I know he's happy.

"She's extraordinary," he says. "She served in Krajina and Kosovo. She's with the firemen."

"Pleasure, ma'am! But you've gotta go now. They may bomb us again."

I have to obey the order. I can't embrace Marko again. He'll reproach me if I do for making a display of affection before his commanding officer. I return to the fire engine, which is ready to go back. The Ministry of Foreign Affairs of Serbia and the DBO (Internal Affairs) buildings are still in flames.

The return trip is arduous, too. Tears sting my eyes and throat. Waves of dust surge through the fire engine's broken passenger-side windows. We often can't even see each other. I'm coughing and trying to hold back my tears. The more I rub my eyes, the worse it gets. We don't have gas masks or oxygen. The firemen have protective helmets, but that's all. I have nothing. I'm learning the hard way. It was thoughtless of me to go out without any safety gear. Now I understand how difficult it is for them to go into flaming buildings after each wave of bombardment.

The fire captain is suffering from severe shoulder pain, but I can't help him in the field. I suggest that he have an X-ray taken, but he shrugs it off.

"Not until we put out these fires," he says, and he immediately continues coordinating the efforts in the area.

"Avala 552, we need a vehicle at the Ministry of Internal Affairs ASAP."

"Avala 550 calling Avala 552. Vehicle from Obrenovac heading your way…."

The vehicles coordinate like bees in a hive. The fireman is grimacing with pain as he holds his radio receiver. Near the Internal Affairs building, we see something moving under a pile of earth and rubble. It's a security guard who was on duty when the building was hit. The debris came tumbling down and buried him. The firemen dig into the debris with shovels and bare hands until the begrimed guard finally emerges. He shakes off the dirt as he coughs and clears his throat. Unlike the guard who was stationed in front of the Ministry of Foreign Affairs, this guy survived. There's a blaze burning right behind him. The firemen lay down track so that the fire engine can get its hoses as close as possible to the flames. The tracks bend and groan beneath the wheels of the truck, but it manages to get close enough. Jets of pressurized water begin dousing the blaze. Soon, the fire engine empties its water tank, but the fire is still burning. As one fire engine departs, another is already moving into position.

A. L. is giving the orders:

"Avala 552, fill your tank at the Mostar Cloverleaf. Avala 552…," says the fire captain, repeating this order several times.

He's grimacing with pain but he's staying on the job. I like this guy.

Something explodes nearby. The blast first deafens me, then knocks me to the ground. My eyes and mouth are filled with dust. My forehead hits rubble, and I feel a sharp, spearing pain travel up my spine. I lie on the ground completely disorientated.

Someone is shaking my shoulders, shouting: "Come on, Doc. Get up! You don't want to be on your knees before NATO. That's what they want, so up you go!"

I manage to get up. Then I realize that I'm not hurt. It's not worth mentioning my bruises or how dirty I am. I spit the dust out of my mouth. We're blackened by dirt and grime. The moment the missile exploded, it flashed through my mind that this was the third cruise missile Marko and General Vukadinović were speaking of. I'm wondering what happened to them. When I'm on my feet again, A. L. tells me that it was not a missile; it was just the old DBO building collapsing, instead. After having already been damaged by a previous missile, the rest has now collapsed. It was a storage depot for the MUP, which is located just behind SUP's Health Center on Durmitorska Street. It falls like a house of cards. I'm relieved when I hear the news because I now know that Marko's safe. We return to the vehicle to shelter ourselves from rolling waves of dust that are now engulfing us. When things calm down, G. P., the driver, starts complaining about the back pain he's experiencing. He and the other guys have already been hurled into the air by an explosion. They were standing beside the fire engine when the first cruise missile hit Army Headquarters, and then the second one lashed them with its tail, whose thrust overturned several vehicles. The fire engine lost its side windows on the driver and passenger sides, but the windshield miraculously remained intact, although it is cracked. After they were thrown by the blast, A. L. landed on his shoulder. He's feeling the pain now. G. L. landed on his back. He says it didn't hurt at first, but now he has trouble walking. You can see the pain on his face. I can't examine him because it's too painful for him to change his position. I asked him if his legs are numb. He says no. I ask if he could breathe normally and he says yes, but his back pain is severe.

"Are your pants dry?" I ask, simply to check his sphincter function.

"You think I shit in my pants 'cause I was scared!?" he retorts angrily.

"No," I say, reassuring him. "Not because you were afraid but because of your injuries. Unfortunately, I can't do much without an X-ray. You have to be examined. The hospital's just round the corner."

"Not yet!" the guys answer in unison.

The fireman sitting next to me is breathing rapidly and moaning quietly, then he cries out in pain.

"I have a pain here in my chest," he wails.

He takes my hand and presses it to his chest. I look at him through the haze of dust and I see a pale gray face with oversized, wide-open eyes. He's trembling. His pulse is rapid, but not excessively so. Maybe he's just scared. He tells me that he fell on the left side of his body. I immediately think that his spleen may have been injured. I ask him to describe precisely where he feels the pain. His explanation is vague, so I ask him to get out of the vehicle so that he can lie down on the asphalt where I can palpate his stomach. I discover that his abdomen is soft, but that's not a definitive sign that his spleen hasn't been damaged. An ultrasound can eliminate that possibility. We simply have to get to the hospital but these guys don't want to go yet, so I just have to doctor them with my hands and my intuition. Another fireman starts venting. He releases an uncontrollable torrent of words.

"I've had it! I give up. I'm a defense engineer — not a fireman. I'm completely covered with dust and I'm dying a couple of times each night. There comes a point when you just say enough is enough. I can just drop dead of stress. My heart can just stop. That can happen any time, right? You're a doctor. Level with me. I could just drop dead of stress, right?"

I could tell him he's absolutely right, but I have the feeling he doesn't want to hear that just now. He doesn't need the truth; he needed encouragement.

"Come on, you don't die just like that!" I say, trying relieve the unbearable tension. "If your number was up, you'd have been dead already. After all, you flew through the air with the greatest of ease and then made a hard landing on your left side. So, no wonder you feel lousy! We'll check you out at the hospital and see how serious it is."

"Ow, it hurts like hell!" he wails. "I can't breathe. Something is making it hard to breathe. Owww! It was awful. There was an explosion and we all went flying, and then we crashed on the pavement. I can still feel it. Feels like my brain turned inside my head. When we got up, the intersection was a disaster. Soldiers were lying dead and wounded in the street. The guard house — well, that disappeared. It went up in smoke. Behind us, a metal bus shelter was heaved up out of the ground and the falling debris severed the legs of that guy you saw at the Medical Center. I never saw so much blood in my life! It was a real massacre. Jesus Christ, when I think of his severed legs lying on the asphalt — still twitching…!"

He pauses. Now he's staring blankly into space.

"We called an ambulance, but they didn't wanna come. Then a military ambulance shows up a couple of minutes later, and they gather up the victims in no time flat. O, God! I can't take this anymore!"

The accumulated tension is blowing his gasket, so he goes on and on. Meanwhile, I see that he's standing in a pool of blood. I'm sure that if he were aware this, his nerves would have snapped.

A couple of unmarked cars with no license plates emerge from the darkness and come to a stop in front of us. A short, balding man emerges from the first car. I recognize him as the man to whom I had complained about the transportation of the wounded when I returned from Kosovo.

The fireman immediately stops his tirade, resumes his professional demeanor, and joins the new arrivals.

"This way, please," he says. "Please, watch out for the rubble."

His retransformation into an efficient fireman takes place in matter of seconds as he disappears into the darkness along with the others.

The light of the full moon barely penetrates the dust cloud. Soon, another fire engine arrives with a group of enthusiastic young men clad red uniforms. We hear the newcomers' laughter through the dim and dusty light.

"Ha ha! You're safe and sound!" shouts their boss.

"They're injured," I call out. "They have to go to the hospital. Each one of 'em's got a problem."

"Let's get you to the hospital," the boss says, still shouting. "This ain't over yet. Where're the others? How many were injured?"

We make a list of the injured on a scrap of wrapping paper from my equipment bag. Everyone is going to be okay. No one is seriously hurt. Most of them are just banged up and bruised. Then the fireman who launched the tirade re-emerges from the shadows.

"How is this guy, Doc?" asks the boss.

"He's my little coward," I say, laughing. "I hope he won't get mad at me for calling him that."

"I doubt it. He's our mascot. He's a radiation expert, so he's one of the first to go into the ruins. You gotta have nerves of steel to do that. He's laying his life on the line."

The crew turns to leave as abruptly as they came.

"Let's get going. There's plenty more work to do," shouts the boss. "We'll see you after your check-ups."

They jump into the fire engine and disappear across a pile of rubble in the direction of the Gazelle Bridge. That part of the street is in complete ruins. Buildings on both sides of the street are smoldering. It's bizarre. I've been in those buildings many times. Now they're burning rubble. The DBO building looks eerily squashed with its double glass walls bulging outward. Toxic, radioactive dust is clinging to my clothing. We don't have gas masks, so I'm completely unprotected. I warn the others to speak as little as possible and to breathe through their noses. A fire breaks out in a metal structure that has collapsed, which is blocking access to the area, but the crew doesn't have a circular to cut through it. We drive to Topčider to get one. The sun is rising; the moon is fading. NATO bombers flee the daylight just as vampires do, and they vanish.

We get the circular saw and we're on our way back to the DBO when we pass the Psychiatric Hospital and the OB Clinic. Both have plenty of windows blown out. I wonder how the psychiatric patients, the mothers awaiting delivery, and the newborns are faring. They're probably still hunkering down by candlelight in the unheated basement to which they've been evacuated.

We deliver the circular saw to the crew. Then we see that gasoline is leaking from our tank. In the morning light, we also get a better look at each other. I suddenly feel the cold and begin trembling. A fireman takes off his jacket and throws it over my shoulders. It's so heavy that I feel like I'm going to fall over. I become dizzy and nauseous, but I'm too embarrassed to faint in the presence of the firemen. After all, I'm the one who's supposed to get them to the Medical Center. We finally reach the Emergency Room, where my colleagues are waiting. Their indistinct faces swarm before my eyes. I'm about to collapse. My skin is irritated and I have trouble breathing. I'm worried about the dust and glass particles we've all inhaled.

"O, you're radioactive! And you've got toxic burns!" exclaims one of my colleagues, who comes running up to me. "Go to detox, right now!"

"I'll manage," I say. "Take care of the firemen, especially the pale guy here. He might be bleeding internally."

Goran, the anesthetist from my department, embraces me.

"What happened to Marko?" he then asks.

"He's all right," I say. "But members of his security detail were killed. He escaped by the skin of his teeth. Goran, I'm so, so tired."

Goran takes me to the clinic and leaves me in the bathroom. There, another nurse helps me take a bath and detoxify. Water is poured over me to wash off the radioactive contamination. They hook me up to an IV, and the infusion begins flowing into me. I have to get rid of all the toxins. I'll feel better in a couple of hours — much better. I can then get some rest, but I just can't fall asleep. My skin is still burning.

Marko arrives later. He was at the VMA where his companions have already been operated on. They weren't in such bad shape, but they did need to undergo surgery. No reason for me to panic now. Marko is alive. We're both alive.

28. Trauma Is Life and Life Is Trauma

May 10, 1999

Yesterday was May 9, the day we celebrate our Victory against Fascism during World War II. Had we really been victorious? Pity the children growing up today. Their childhoods have been traumatized. Ljuba, my younger daughter, gets a panic attack whenever she hears sirens. First she cries, then she screams. Marija, the eldest, is afraid to fall asleep. She just lies awake —

as if there's some difference between being killed awake instead of asleep.

NATO bombed Niš in broad daylight. They dropped cluster bombs — forbidden weapons — into an open-air market full of people, where they killed a pregnant woman as well as an elderly woman, whose shopping bag and its contents were scattered beside her body. NATO claims that their missiles are exclusively targeting key military installations, but they're also killing and maiming children.

May 17, 1999

I feel terrible. I've been exposed to radioactive dust. The cruise missile that struck near my hospital in Belgrade was highly radioactive. The Geiger counter readings were going off the chart. The radioactivity levels around the Ministry of Foreign Affairs, the Ministry of Internal Affairs, and the IT buildings are also much higher than any permissible levels. *NATO is planning to kill us now by bombardment, and then later — slowly, very slowly — by radioactive contamination.*

My skin was spotted — as if I had chicken pox. Small blisters appeared, then quickly dried up. My skin is now peeling. I look terrible. My lungs feel like they're failing. I have to take asthma medication. I suffer from diarrhea. I can barely leave the toilet. The Medical Center doesn't have a detoxification chamber. I have no experience with radioactive contamination, but I'm getting it now — and how!

Yesterday, I went to Smederevo to see my children, as well as to pick up a letter that I received by registered mail from who knows where. The children aren't steady on their feet yet. They're frustrated and full of hatred for the invisible war planes of faraway countries — whose citizens don't really care enough to go out into the streets and protest against the bombardment. This feeling of helplessness my children feel is only going to ripen — if we survive all this — into outright contempt and hatred. This experience isn't going to do us any good. I'm not sure what kind of people we're going to turn into. We're just going to have to live with contempt and hatred. How can we forgive the world? We mustn't forgive. If we do, they will continue to act tyrannically and kill with impunity whenever they wish. That's what I'm afraid of: a global policemen who has absolute power and authority to act as judge, jury, and executioner.

I'm sleeping with the children now for the first time since the bombardment began. Our sleep is light and brief. Distant explosions and anti-aircraft defense fire keep waking us up. Marija says it's good to hear explosions that are far away because she thinks there's nothing to worry about — for the time being. We visit a neighbor whose brother-in-law was injured during a missile attack. He was lucky. He survived. A friend who was with him was killed. Our apartment is near the Kovin Bridge, which has also been destroyed. People resort to using ferries to cross the Danube, just as they did up until a hundred years ago. It's the same in Novi Sad where the Army set up a pontoon bridge that spans the river banks, and which temporarily enables transportation.

I followed Adem's advice. In January 1999, I learned on the Internet that Norway does, indeed, need one thousand doctors. If they need that many doctors, then there surely has to be a place for me. So I wrote to Professor Gisvold in Trondheim. He was the moderator at the World Congress on Resuscitation that was held in Copenhagen in 1998. I presented three scientific papers there, one of which I presented orally. I didn't know whether he remembered me, but it was worth trying to contact him. I wrote him an emotional letter asking for help in finding a position. A Norwegian language professor later advised me that I had used an inappropriate tone. Well, you can't unring the bell after it's been rung, and besides, I don't want to change either myself or my style. I'm an emotional being, and I don't have any intention of hiding it. The Professor answered in what turned out to be an uncharacteristic Norwegian style. He said that he had forwarded my letter to five nearby hospitals in the area where he lives. He wants to help, and he hopes that I'll find a job in one of them. He wishes me luck. I don't suppose that he has any idea of what this means to me. After having experienced so much tragedy in Serbia, I finally feel that my own private sun is going to rise, and that it's going to shine only for me. I zealously begin learning Norwegian.

The registered letter I got turned out to be from Norway. A hospital in Kristiansund requested my *curriculum vitae* along with various personal documents and two references with phone numbers. They acknowledged receiving a recommendation letter from Professor E. Gisvold, and they advised me that they had a vacant position they wanted to fill.

With all this chaos going on, how do I get references and how can I possibly send the necessary documents?

May 25, 1999

Today is Ljuba's birthday. She's twelve. She's in Smederevo. I'm in Belgrade — stuck in the clinic. I can't even give her a hug today. My nerves are on edge. The world is imprisoning us in our own country.

May 28, 1999

Today, a directive arrives advising me that I have to go to Kosovo in the next few days. Where in Kosovo? Why me again? I feel that I've already reached the outer limits of exhaustion. I have no motivation whatsoever to go there again. I try to find out why they chose me — me again! — out of the thousand anesthesiologists in Serbia. No one can give me an answer.

June 3, 1999

Yesterday, Yugoslavia signed the terms of surrender. After seventy-eight days of constant bombardment, and after seventy-eight sleepless nights, a night finally arrived when we could sleep without sirens and without invisible war planes bombing us. I have no comment. One catastrophe is over — but I don't know what's coming next.

June 12, 1999

Today, I set out for Kosovo with two other doctors. We're supposed to go to Peć. The driver who came to pick us up in Belgrade told us that a nurse in Peć had informed him that the Albanian authorities decided (behind closed doors) to dismiss the entire hospital staff. The three of us are told to wait for new orders, but we were further advised that the mission wasn't going to be canceled. I don't understand what the problem is, but I'm happy go home.

Meanwhile, I received news that the Andrejević Charitable Foundation is going to hold a book promotion on June 17 at the Ethnographic Museum. My doctoral dissertation on the subject of fear and stress in anesthesia was accepted in an open competition, and then it was chosen as the best among the top ten finalists. I revised and expanded my thesis, which resulted in a book, *Fear and Anesthesia*. I'm looking forward to the event. The bombing hasn't crushed us, after all.

June 15, 1999

This afternoon, a colleague advises me that the Ministry of Health called. The Ministry said I was going to Kosovo in the morning. I get a call from the managing director of the Medical Center, too. Why am I going to Kosovo now? Aren't the Serbs leaving Kosovo in droves before the Albanians, who are burning and destroying everything in their path, sweep through? The

KLA is running wild but KFOR is doing nothing to rein them in. I'm supposed to leave tomorrow. What about the book promotion? I run to the Administration Building of the Medical Center to see the managing director. I tell him I can't go. I explain to him that the promotion of this — my second book — is important to me.

"Postpone the promotion!" he demands, insisting on getting his way.

"What other time? A charitable foundation is hosting the promotion. I can't do anything about it. I'm very happy to have this book promotion — even at a crazy time like this. There's no chance of postponing it," I say, pleading.

"That's none of my business," he says indifferently. "You have to go, and nothing should prevent you from going. This book promotion is just incidental. In any case, you'll be fired if you don't go."

He dismisses me. I'm dumbfounded by his arrogance. He then turns his back and leaves. There are one thousand anesthesiologists in Serbia, a hundred and twenty-four in the Medical Center of Serbia alone, and he's sending me to Kosovo under the threat of losing my job? What the hell is that supposed to mean? I call Marko and tell him everything. But he's a soldier, so he doesn't know how to protest an order.

"Never mind," he says. "We'll organize the promotion somehow without you. Calm down. You've got a job offer in Norway. It would be best for you to fulfill this obligation. You've been in worse situations. And just think! After that, you'll be free to do whatever you want. Remember, you've got a chance to get out of here. The rest of us don't."

That's true. I got a job offer in Kristiansund, Norway.

I call Ksenija Jovanović, the distinguished actress from the National Theater in Belgrade. She's a friend who supported my efforts to present the other side of war, so she agrees to read my acceptance speech at the event.

The next day, thirty of us set out for Kosovo in two cars and a minibus while the inhabitants of Kosovo are leaving. We're going against an endless line of poor people who are driving tractors loaded with luggage and household possessions. I saw similar columns of refugees back in Krajina in 1991, and again in 1995 when two hundred thousand of the last Serbs in Croatia drove, ran, and walked to Serbia. Now a similar column of refugees is fleeing Kosovo. It's heartbreaking to see the disheveled and disorganized members of paramilitary forces who joined this column. But we're going *to* Kosovo. Who are we going to treat there, anyway?

Our drivers are nervous because it's difficult negotiating the overcrowded roads. From time to time, we get stuck in a traffic jam so we end up waiting for fifteen, twenty, thirty minutes just to get moving again. The roads have been torn up and the bridges bombed, so we have to take detours across antiquated bridges that creak under the weight of our vehicles. People, some armed, others not, were emerging from the forest. It's dangerous along these roads. We finally arrive at a motel near Raška, where we stop. The motel has been damaged by the bombardment. Almost all its windows are broken.

Our convoy simply can't go any further, so we have lunch in a nearby restaurant. The main road has been obstructed by large cisterns. The police are trying to stop the great column of people who are leaving Kosovo. They're forcing people to return, just as in 1995 when the police were forcing refugees from Krajina on the roads to Serbia back into the jaws of the enemy.

At the motel, a long line has already formed for the only available telephone, which is at the reception desk. We get in line. I want to call Marko to learn how the book promotion went. Staff members from the Priština hospital, who had fled, are also in line. They're running for their lives. They're lucky because they can stay with relatives in Serbia. Most of them have already left. No more than 300 of the 1,500 members of the hospital staff remain. First, the Albanian staff disappeared, so everyone knows something's up; the Albanians are surely planning to take over the hospital by force. In that case, who's going to protect the Serbs now that the Army has left? And who's going to protect these people that the police are forcing back into Kosovo?

"The Albanians are setting fire to everything and they're killing everyone," the women in line warn us.

She continues intently.

"We're all fleeing in panic. No one's going to help us. You're crazy to go there. What do you think you're going to do there? And what's going to happen to the hospital after it falls into the hands of the Albanians?"

"What'll happen to the Serbian staff that stays in the hospital?" we ask.

"Who knows? They know you can't help them. You'll just be a burden. The hospital can't function with only 20% of its staff. Besides, the enemy has it surrounded and it's cutting off all supplies of food and medicine."

The nurses from Priština elaborate further, so we all know that our journey has become pointless. There's no prudent course of action left for us to take, so our team becomes sullen and withdrawn. I manage to get Marko on the phone, and while he's telling me about the book promotion, I suddenly lose interest. He goes on talking without realizing that I want to change the subject. The people in line behind me are nervous and they keep interrupting me. I hang up without telling him how worried I am that we might never see each other again.

One of my colleagues telephones the hospital staff in Priština. They're still inside the hospital, but Albanian forces are already outside just waiting to take it over. I stand in line for the telephone again. I call Saša on his cell phone and try to persuade him to leave Kosovo with the remaining staff. Serbs can't remain there without suffering serious losses. Why risk so many lives? Alive they can leave; dead, they stand no chance. Saša connects me with the acting Hospital Director, an orthopedist named Rade Grbić. I tell him of the difficulties we're encountering on our way, and what people coming from Kosovo are telling us. I also tell him that there's little chance that we'll reach the hospital alive. And even if we do, what are we going to do then? He's realistic. He realizes everything is already hopeless. He says that he will give the matter some more thought.

The driving rain sweeps through the broken windows and into our room. Soon the beds are soaking wet, so we aren't going to be able to sleep here. We go back outside, where we learn there is a bus station behind the motel. It's full of agitated and panic-stricken people. There are some 500 children in one place and they're all bawling at the top of their lungs. We return to the motel and ask the receptionist if we can let the children in because it's cold and raining outside.

"No!" the motel manager replies curtly.

He says there are too many and that the motel can't put them all up. "If we let them in," adds the front desk clerk, "then the others will pile in behind them along with all the criminals. Then we'll have a stampede. That's all we need!"

The main road is a short distance away, but it has been log jammed by a column of tractors, cars, and vehicles drawn by dray animals. It is the second day of the exodus from Kosovo. These people are hungry, but no one is providing them with food. We brought a lot of food because we knew from previous experience that it was going to be difficult to come by, so we go back to the motel and we bring out all the food we've got. Our arms were full. We tread carefully down the stairs to avoid tripping and falling. We divide ourselves into groups. We speak in hushed tones. The tension is becoming unbearable. An anesthesiologist polls our group, and he learns that the others also want to return to Belgrade. Outside, I speak to our escort from the Ministry of Health. I suggest that we return home. They shake their heads and tell us that they will advise us of the revised plans in the morning at nine. No one can sleep. In the morning, relentless columns of refugees from Kosovo are working their way toward Serbia. How are we going travel in the opposite direction against this rising tide of dispossessed refugees?

And who's going to drive us back to Belgrade? Our escort is coming back but my nervous colleagues are now upset. Several declare that they are returning to Belgrade immediately. How are they going to do that? The roads are dangerous. We can get ourselves killed by traveling in either direction. There isn't much of a difference between getting killed by either Albanian or Serbian criminals. We have to calm down and stick together.

"If we go to Priština, you're going to have to go ahead of us," I say to our escort. "If you disagree, then we're all going back to Belgrade together."

"No, we could get killed," he says.

"If they kill you, then they'll kill us too," I insist.

"You aren't as important to the government as we are," he says, demeaning me.

"Are you out of your mind?" I shoot back. "How can you possibly consider yourself more important than thirty people? It's just as I told you: either you're driving ahead of us or we're all going back to Belgrade. There's no other way. We're all going together in either one or the other direction. And I demand the protection of the UN."

"I'm arresting you in the name of the government of the Republic of Serbia as the traitor to the Serbian people," says one of the escorts.

Waking Up to a New Struggle

He was serious. He was an Albanian from the Serbian Ministry of Health. He seized both my hands. I felt dizzy. An Albanian was arresting me as a traitor to the Serbian people because I'm not foolish enough to get myself killed!? My eyes narrowed in disbelief as he tightened his grip as if he were about to handcuff me. A hot flash hit my head, and then everything went red before my eyes. I fainted. I felt as if I were falling. The Albanian was still holding my wrists in his vise-like grip, while his malicious laughter was echoing in the darkness subsuming me.

"I thought you were a brave woman, but now I see that you're just a coward!"

Those were the last words I heard.

I couldn't remember anything at all after that until I regained consciousness in my mother's apartment. My children were sitting at the edge of my bed. What was I doing here? I was unable to speak. My tongue was swollen. What happened to me? I wanted to get up but I couldn't. Out of the corner of my eye, I saw my mother wiping tears from her eyes. Why was she crying? Why was I in her apartment instead of in my own apartment or Marko's? I wanted to ask her but I was unable to express myself. The telephone rang. My eldest daughter got up, answered, and told someone on the other end of the line that I had regained consciousness but that I was unable to speak. Who was she talking to? I wanted to scream and warn her not to tell anyone anything — absolutely nothing! These are dangerous times.

I lay in bed for days. I was unable to get up by myself. My daughters and my mother assisted me when I had to use the toilet. They forced me to eat even though I had a lot of difficulty swallowing food. I had a persistent headache. Tears were blurring my vision.

Two weeks later, I was able to stand on my feet again, albeit unsteadily. The teary vision suddenly ended. My daughters were beside me. What had happened to me? From time to time, ambulance drivers from Belgrade came to our house. Their faces and voices were familiar but I couldn't remember where I knew them from. It was already July. Almost a month had passed since the bombardment ended. I was half-asleep for most of the month. It was all because of stress. I remembered being arrested, but I still didn't know how I had gotten home or what had happened to the others in the group.

A colleague who had been on the trip visited me. He said that I was "arrested" after I had expressed my opposition to continuing the trip to Kosovo. Then I fainted. So, we were all saved because I had lost consciousness. They put me in a car and wasted no time driving me back to Belgrade. Once they arrived, the others went their separate ways and didn't say a word about the incident. They didn't want to be arrested. I was accommodated at home instead of at the hospital for fear that I too might be arrested. Frightened colleagues called my mother and asked her to urge me not to publicize the incident. I was unable to speak, and, needless to say, I was incapable of dealing with the media. I couldn't understand why I felt this way. Was I really so vulnerable? Did this experience crush me? I've been through a lot since 1990. All this could have finally taken its toll.

I learned that my colleagues in Priština left the hospital immediately upon our return to Belgrade. They took only the most necessary personal belongings and left Kosovo in their own private cars. The hospital, and all the equipment in which Serbia had invested so much, was abandoned. The Albanians simply commandeered it for their own exclusive use. The same thing happened to all the other hospitals in Kosovo.

I couldn't bear listening to these stories any more. The most important thing was that they had all survived. Meanwhile, I was still suffering from a persistent headache, which was contributing to my blurred vision. After an uncontrollable flood of tears, it flashed through my mind that Marko hadn't yet come to visit me. Days passed, but he still wasn't calling or inquiring about me. It was strange. Did something happened to him? I couldn't ask my mother or my children. They already had enough problems taking care of me.

On July 8, I get a CT scan in an ambulance. Since I'm unable to move my left arm and my left leg, it's clear that my illness involves more than just stress. My power of speech is slowly returning. I can speak slowly, but I often have trouble finding the right words.

I'm looking at the X-rays from the CT scan with the radiographer when a radiologist, whom I've known since my university days, arrives. She embraces me warmly. She doesn't realize that she's looking at an X-ray of *my* brain. She studies the image, evaluates it, and says:

"A massive cerebral infarction in the right hemisphere. The patient is probably paralyzed on the left side and unable to speak. Look, it extends as far as —"

Then she stops in the middle of the sentence.

That's what happened to me, I realize at that moment. *I suffered a stroke.*

"Whose X-ray is this?" she asks cautiously.

"It's Dr. Mitic's!" says a neurosurgeon who has arrived in the meantime.

"I'm sorry! I'm sorry I didn't know," she sputters nervously. "I thought that you were here for a consultation about another patient. What happened? Aren't you the one who had the accident in Kosovo? You'll recover; you're young. You're alive! The brain very quickly recovers from collateral damage. Just practice and practice. I'm not worried about you. You've always been full of energy. You're going to overcome this."

Tears come to their eyes, which is harder for me to take than my condition. Well, if I have to rehabilitate myself, then that's just what I'm going to do!

On our way back home, I ask the ambulance driver to take me to Belgrade's City Hall. I want to find out what happened to Marko. I don't have the strength to get out of the car, so I send my colleague from the hospital who's accompanying me to ask Marko to come outside and say hello, but he returns to tell me that Marko can't come just now. He says he'll call me later.

I'm shocked and dismayed. After all that we had gone through together, he wasn't even going to come out to say hello. No, no, I think, reconsidering. Maybe I shouldn't look at it that way. I don't really understand what's keeping him from coming out to see me — but it's still painful.

"Who's he?" asks my colleague, who was also on that fateful journey to Kosovo, when he realizes that I'm offended.

"Hmm! I'm trying to remember," I answer, dodging the question. "You know I probably suffered brain damage!"

I try to make light of it, but he stops the car. He embraces me.

"Forget about him," he says. "He's not worth it. We, who are alive today thanks to you, are profoundly grateful. We all could have been killed. I dread to think of it. Let's just put it behind us."

After work, Marko comes to my mother's apartment. I'm asleep, so I didn't hear the doorbell. My mother tries to send him away because she doesn't want to see him. His absence in my most difficult moments is a sure sign that he doesn't really care much about me. I'm of the same opinion, but I don't want her to meddle in my affairs. Sick and unsteady on my feet, I still manage to get up and invite him in. Then I have it out with him. There is simply no justification for his conduct, although he tries to justify himself by saying that he's just afraid of losing his job; that he's going to lose everything again; that he's not going to be able to help me. Maybe it's true, maybe it's not. But surely no one would have held it against him if he had stepped out of the office to say hello to an old friend who was sick, an old friend whom he supposedly loved.

I inherited a memory filter from my mother, so I can excise, without anesthesia, one part of myself and still continue living. I regenerate myself like a hydra. My attitude is that we can continue living without looking back. That's the only way you can survive after a traumatic experience. I don't know whether these ghosts from the past will ambush me at some unexpected moment in the future, but now I realize that I have to live without some aspects of my former self.

Two days later, my brother drove me home and left me with my daughters. I had headaches nearly every day, so I wasn't even tempted to think about what happened. My apartment in Smederevo is a mess after my three-month absence. Thanks to the bombardment, it had a new set of broken windows. I cleaned the apartment room by room with my daughters' help. It was slow going. I was unsteady on my feet. My head was swimming, and I couldn't see straight because of the migraine headaches. I had to start doing something — anything — a hundred times before I could finish it. My girls took me for a walk twice a day, before sunrise and after sunset, to the Smederevo Fortress. I tried to fit regular exercise into my daily routine. At first, my girls had to hold me by either arm as I slowly walked. Soon, I began moving faster and faster. In the beginning, I exercised for an hour each day; later, I was able to exercise for longer periods of time. I grew stronger by the day. I didn't watch television. I didn't talk about what had happened. I tried to forget. My neighbors helped a great deal. Their sense of humor kept me going.

One day, a registered package arrived from Norway. It was hefty. It probably contained the documents I had submitted that were now being returned to me. I didn't have enough strength to withstand another disappointment, so I dumped the unopened package into the trash.

"What if they're offering you a job?" asked my daughter.

"No, that's impossible," I said. "Who'd hire me? I'm unfit for duty."

My daughters were more curious than I was. Ljuba retrieved the package and opened it. It didn't contain the documents that I had submitted; instead, it contained beautiful brochures describing a quaint island town. Strange winding roads went up and down crags that beetled over the sea. Three beautiful bridges linked the island to the mainland. I tried to imagine what would have happened if NATO had bombed these bridges as they had bombed ours. Could these people have managed — ? O, my! Why am I thinking this way?

Among the many illustrated brochures describing the city and the hospital, there was a letter inviting me to visit the Fylkesjykehuset in Kristinasund (The Kristiansund County Hospital). I was supposed to contact the head of the department by the middle of August in order to make arrangements for my visit. Conflicting thoughts besieged me. Why do I need this? I'm crippled, paralyzed. And I can barely speak. I forgot all the Norwegian I had learned. I can only read English and there's no chance of me speaking it. I'm useless.

During one of my walks with my daughters, I sat down on a park bench and cried.

Finally, my daughters set me straight: "Mom, enough's enough! You taught us that life is no fairy tale. Get up and fight! Stop crying or soon we're going to be the laughing stock of the whole town!"

Once we got home, we carefully reviewed all the material I had received. The invitation to visit raised my spirits and rekindled my energy. God wouldn't have given me a second chance if I had been unable to live up to it. I exercised every morning and evening at the Smederevo Fortress, which became my faithful friend. Its mighty, centuries-old ramparts filled me with energy. My feeble legs were soon walking faster. The wind caressed my face. I could hear the voices of those who built this fortress with the last atom of their strength in order to protect Serbia from the Ottoman invasion. Their hands now rose out of the past and urged me forward. I began to think about the future again. I started studying Norwegian again. I took large quantities of analgesics to ease my headaches. Sometimes tears welled up in my eyes, but I don't pay any attention to them anymore.

29. The Secret of My Origins

The decision to leave Serbia is inevitable but difficult. Everything I own and everyone I love is here. I have to break with the past and head into the unknown. It isn't easy. Before I left, I sold my apartment along with everything in it. People have no money. No one was interested in buying an apartment as an investment. The buyers would probably be refugees from Kosovo or from other parts of the former Yugoslavia. This apartment had cost me a great deal of effort. To me, it was a living being, so I couldn't just leave it to strangers. Over the years, I furnished it with things that I loved that are now disappearing from my life. Some paintings and other valuables I just gave away to my friends. Many of them had helped me along my arduous journey in life, so I wanted to show them my gratitude and appreciation. Besides, it was easier to leave treasured possessions with people whose friendship I cherished. I love art, which explains why there weren't any empty spaces on my walls. Now these paintings are going to grace the walls of my friends' homes. My apartment was a symbol of personal safety just as it was an expression of victory over the system. It's all beginning to fade away.

I sold the flat to the parents of a fellow anesthesiologist I worked with. They wanted to move from the village into the city to be closer to their grandchildren. They didn't have the money to meet my asking price, so I lowered it. I was satisfied. I'll never forget his mother's surprised exclamation. She loved the apartment, so I was delighted. When I closed the door for the last time, I could still see the spray-painted cross with *1994* written beneath it. I wasn't able to remove it, so it remained as a reminder of what had happened to Miroslav.

My daughters and I visited his grave once again to pay our respects to his memory. We hadn't forgotten him. How could we have? People we have known and loved occupy a special place in our lives. I began saying good-bye to everyone I could find.

I once had a patient, Vera, whom I remember as a medical miracle. She had spinal surgery without anesthetics, of which she had a life-long fear. When she needed to have surgery a second time, she refused to go to the hospital until she met with me. I have a Ph.D. in anesthesia, and I took my Master's Degree in Psychosomatic Illnesses. With my additional interest in Psychology, I was the right person to help her, but it was not as simple a task as I had hoped. She didn't fall asleep on the operating table even though she had received four adult doses of anesthetics. I was worried that I wasn't going to be able to help her by sticking to standard procedures. But my desire to help solve her problem and get her into surgery inspired me to try hypnosis, even though it is not an accepted treatment method in Serbia. In the end, her operation was successful, and she didn't feel a thing. We were both happy with the outcome. As I was leaving, the hospital, she told me that I wouldn't be living in Serbia for much longer, and that I would be traveling to a far-away country. I didn't pay much attention to what she said. Many would have given all they had for an opportunity to leave, and I was one of them. But at the time, I didn't have anywhere to go. Later, when I realized that I was going to be leaving for Norway, I smiled wistfully as I remembered her words.

Just before I left Smederevo for Belgrade, Vera brought presents for me and my children. Among other things, she told me that it was important for me to know that I was not ethnically Serbian, as I had thought and as I had claimed. My family, which emigrated from Russia to the Balkans, had changed its identity. Most of my relatives stayed in the Balkans, but others were scattered all over the world. According to her, my heritage is Jewish.

"My dear Vera, I love and respect you," I said. "But don't expect me to believe what you just told me. I am a Yugoslav who chose to be a Serb. I haven't stopped being a Yugoslav, and now you tell me that my heritage is not Serbian but Jewish! This is too much for my brain to process. At this moment, when I'm on the verge of leaving Serbia–Yugoslavia, I need stability. I have to know who I am and where I'm going. I am not a tree without roots that any gust of wind can topple. I'm sorry, but I'm a Serb. I was born in the capital, where I grew up as a Yugoslav, but after the country disintegrated, I became a Serb. Case closed!"

Vera smiled enigmatically, caressed my cheek, hugged me and left, but her words continued to haunt me. If she hadn't earlier correctly predicted that I would be going abroad, I wouldn't have paid any attention to what she said about my heritage. But her prediction was now coming true. So, after having reconsidered what she had said, I decided that there may, instead, be some truth to her story.

Of course, I consulted my mother. She could tell me if there was any truth to what Vera had said.

As I was telling her about Vera's prediction (or whatever I should call it), tears began rolling down her cheeks. Then she covered her face with her hands and she sobbed inconsolably. Her entire body was convulsing. Frightened, I flung my arms around her and held her.

"What's the matter you? Please, look at me!" I cried.

My children, who witnessed the scene, simply thought that Grandma was crying because we had come to say good-bye because we were leaving for Norway.

My mother stopped crying as suddenly as she had begun. She wiped away her tears, and she asked me to bring her the ring I had received as a gift from her mother. My jewelry was in a separate box that I was going to carry on the plane with me, so the ring was at hand.

I brought it to her. She was now smiling poignantly as she held it in her hands.

"I'm so surprised — it's funny how impossible it is to hide anything in life. You can hide the truth all you want, but sooner or later it's inevitably revealed. God finds ways to open doors so that the truth comes to light. There are many things to which we are blind, especially those that we're concealing, which others may plainly see. In one instance, it may be a hidden document; in another, a lack of insight.

"What are you talking about?" I asked. "What Vera said isn't important."

"That's exactly why it *is* important. She was speaking the truth, a truth I never thought anyone would ever reveal. And knowing you and your inquisitive nature, you might as well know the whole story. So, it's better if we settle this here and now."

"What story? We're Serbs! I'm proud of it, even though it isn't easy being one now. Serbs have suffered just as the Jews have. Serbs lost their country just like the Jews once did."

"Sarah, we are Jews! I am Jewish on my mother's side, just as your father is. We're Jewish, my child!"

"What?!"

A strange weakness overcame me, so I had to sit down and take a deep breath. Everything began to ache. Luminous patches of fireworks were shimmering with color and emotion before my eyes.

My mother showed me the ring my grandmother had chosen to leave to me. It featured three sparkling Stars of David. The inner band bore a Hebrew inscription. This ring has been passed on from generation to generation in our family, from one woman to another. I will give it to one of my daughters for her children's sake.

I held the ring tightly and wept. After I inherited it, I replaced the two blue stones with white ones because people said blue was bad luck. Now I regret having done that. I had no idea of how precious it was. It was a one-hundred-and-fifty-year-old heirloom that bound me to my unknown past.

Since my grandmother passed away, I'm unable to ask her any of the numerous questions I have. My mother can't answer them all. All she inherited was the secret. In order to escape the persecution inflicted upon the Jewish people, my family changed its name. Some relatives even changed their faith. My mother's family lived in Croatia where 700,000 people lost their lives during WWII — over 40,000 of them Jews. If they hadn't been disguised as Serbs, they would have ended up in the Jasenovac Concentration Camp.[21]

After WWII, no one in Croatia was held responsible for the mass murders of Serbs and Jews. No one! That was why my family had decided to keep quiet. They were living among the murderers of relatives and fellow citizens. The Fascists, after the war had turned against them, quickly changed allegiance and transformed themselves into Communist Partizans. My family had to survive. Those who died were forgotten, but the living passed on the genes.

---

21. *Jasenovac Concentration Camp*, an extermination camp established by the Ustaša regime in the Independent State of Croatia during WWII. It was the only concentration camp not operated by the Nazis. It is often referred to as the "Auschwitz of the Balkans." The Simon Wiesenthal Center estimates that 600,000 people were killed there. Other estimates are higher.

And genes cannot be disguised, even if you're clueless to their origin.

I immediately understood why all the women in my family had problems with bleeding. We inherited a typical genetic characteristic of Ashkenazi Jews. I used to wonder how I ended up with this condition. I could have died in childbirth because of this genetic predisposition. God alone saved me from certain death. What else could I have inherited? What else had been hidden from my generation — not to mention earlier generations?

There is no answer. The only thing my mother knew was that we had to look out for one another and conceal our origins. This fear was transmitted from one generation to the next. My grandmother concealed it, but someone exposed her. She was arrested in Croatia during World War II and condemned to death simply because she was Jewish. Luckily, she survived. Her sister, on the other hand, did not. Nor did many of my other relatives.

I can't think about this. We're alive. I understand the message. I have two daughters whom I now have to protect from anti-Semites. What my mother does know is that our ancestors came to the Balkans from St. Petersburg, Russia, most likely during the great persecution of Jews, just as Vera had told me. Images of people waiting in lines — running, screaming, terrified, lost — filled my mind. WWII concentration camps are now a matter of personal history. I feel an uneasy chill, a prelude to trembling.

My mother let me weep silently. She held me and said: "Nothing has changed. You're still the same person you were before you heard this story. Calm down now and focus on the road ahead. There is much that awaits you, and your heritage will only help you. You belong to the world now. Let our Jewish history strengthen you, but let it also instruct you. Be careful and be smart. You have to survive. Life is all important. We kept a secret — but we survived."

I surely had some questions that my mother may not have wished to answer and perhaps couldn't have answered. Why did she and my father keep this hidden — until now? She did mention that my father's mother was Jewish, too. I loved my paternal grandmother immensely, yet I knew nothing about her.

* * * *

I can hear my mother saying:

"You knew only as much as you needed to know. You know what both of your grandmothers were like and you know that they were human beings. What mattered most was that they loved you — and remarkably so.

"I didn't know much about my parents, either, but during the war, I learned how to remain silent. We were living in constant fear of someone arresting or attacking us. The men only wore a kippah in the house behind locked doors. We children couldn't even mention it. Our neighbors didn't work on Sundays, and we didn't work on Saturdays. If asked about it, we said that we were entitled to a day of rest, but God didn't specify which one. During WWII, danger was lurking everywhere. My family was persecuted in Nazi Croatia because they were "Serbs," who themselves didn't have an easier time of it. Even though they outnumbered other nationalities — or perhaps because of it — they were subjected to mass killings. They were killed more often and were brought to Jasenovac in larger numbers than Jews were. Jews were systematically divided from the rest of the population and murdered, often in gas chambers. With Serbian names, we had a better chance of survival than Jews — who had none.

"The Serbs were organized and they defended themselves. They are fighters and they had already had bad experiences with their Croatian neighbors. The Jews were caught off guard. They didn't really believe that they would be killed because they knew that they had done nothing to merit such violence. Maybe that's why they neither fought back nor joined the Serbs to fight the

Fascists. We survived the war, but then we had to pay tribute to the Communists. They could be just as evil and cruel as the Nazis were. Problems dogged our family, but we didn't have time to concentrate on anything except survival. The Balkans have always been turbulent and dangerous.

"During the post-war period, the truth surfaced about how many Jews had been killed. Awful stories and even shocking photos came to light. Tito's allies in Yugoslavia — Croats, Bosnian Muslims, Albanians — had been the perpetrators, and now they were the very same people with whom we were co-existing in the spirit of *brotherhood and unity*. But no one punished the Croats or the Bosnian Muslims or the Albanians who had sided with Hitler. They went scot free. After the war, everyone ganged up on the Serbian anti-Communists, the only people who had protected us from the Nazis long before the Communist Partisans ever arrived on the scene.

"It's probably hard for you to understand, but the fear never went away, even during Tito's rule. *He* allowed the Nazi collaborators to go unpunished, and *he* allowed them to join the Communist Party. Your father and I were frightened by our own shadows. In 1948, your father was arrested, tarred, and driven around Belgrade with his friends on top of a car screaming: *Tito or Stalin? Tito or Stalin?*

"Your father had been permanently disabled during the war. He repeated wildly: *Tito is ours! Tito is ours!"*

"After that, your father was declared a Communist. He was exemplary, always the best, always the first one to arrive at work and the last one to leave. You know he was seldom home during your childhood.

"His friends were in shock but they couldn't say a word. Otherwise, they would have been taken to Goli Otok to be killed.[22] 150,000 people ended up there. Tito had all of his opponents murdered there. That was how he destroyed the Serbian intelligentsia, which was largely anti-Communist.

"As I said, your father had a strong work ethic, which we passed on to you. You were an extraordinary student — at the top of your class. You were and still are energetic and engaged, and you have a passion for justice. You stand out from the rest and that causes envy in others. We were afraid that something might happen to you. You were also a great athlete, but the Neo-Nazi PLO killed eleven Jewish athletes at the Munich Olympics. That frightened us even more, so we knew that our secret had to die with us. Staying quiet and protecting your children from madmen was the best we could do. You were safe living in ignorance. People may be prejudiced despite amiable appearances. They label Jews with visible as well as invisible yellow stars, and whenever anyone put some pressure them, they easily turn against Jews. That's how it has been throughout history. We didn't want you to go through that.

"You did a school project about the Jewish Holocaust in high school. I was devastated when I saw how uneasy you felt as you were choosing the photographs to use for your presentation. I remember how you lamented over their tragic fate, which was the fate of your unknown relatives. Telling you anything at that time would have been wrong. How could I have shared the secret with you since our ancestors wanted to keep it hidden? They wanted their descendants to live in ignorance. Everything was so

---

22. *Goli Otok* is a barren island off the coast of Croatia where political prisoners were imprisoned by the Yugoslav Communists.

complicated, so our heritage was better off as a secret kept by the few of us who knew. Most of our family doesn't know a thing about it.

"A Jewish woman took care of you when you were a child," my mother continued. "Marta, whom you called 'Mitzi', loved you as if you were her own child because she lost her family in the concentration camps. We never told her that we were Jews. She lived with us as a family member and she was surprised by how easily we accepted her Jewish customs. She wanted to return to her faith, so she took you along to the synagogue. But she was unable to identify with the stories of our six-thousand-year-old heritage, so she became disappointed. In any case, she believed that Jews had to be involved in the present and that they had to turn the wheel of society's evolution. Often, she would say that if G–d had named the Jews as His chosen people, then they must be the ones who can discern His intentions. They have been chosen to work more than others, to learn more than others, to shun materialism and to attach themselves instead to the spiritual life. That's what kept them alive throughout history. Material wealth vanishes easily, but knowledge remains until a man dies or is killed. European culture committed suicide by attempting to eradicate the very same Jewish life that helped create Europe.

"G–d gave us the ability to love because love is the greatest manifestation of religious faith. Many a war has shown us what happens when one religion claims the exclusive right to the truth or when one nation steps forward and claims the exclusive right to justice. We Jews must be the link between different religions and nations. These words were part of Mitzi's last will and testament.

"My dear, there are many like you in Serbia who are unaware of their Jewish heritage. This way, they are safer, just as you were. I'm worried because you're much more vulnerable now.

The fate of the Jews in Israel is tragic. They live in constant fear of attack. They're isolated. They have to defend themselves not only in Israel but abroad as well. Sometimes, I get the feeling they voluntarily went into yet another concentration camp, one which anti-Semites can destroy with a single missile. It's not easy living on the edge with your fists clenched all the time, ready to either fight or flee. I'm afraid this same fate awaits you: the continued danger from — as well as the need to protect yourself from — people who believe that Jews are responsible for their own problems and their own failures in life. You'll remember my words after you've had your first conversation with a Jew hater, and there are plenty of them.

"You're asking me whether I raised you to be Jewish, Serbian, or Yugoslav. I raised you to be a good person. Being a good person is of the utmost importance. That's something no one can take away from you. Love is also important. Those who love are capable of creating miracles, and I always wanted my children to procreate and love people. You have, thank the Lord, learned this from your father and me, and if you pass this onto your children, then you will be worthy of our heritage. Then I'll know that I've taught you what other Jews have taught their children, what I learned from my Jewish mother and grandmother. Our fate is to wander the world. You are leaving now. Don't cry for Serbia. You'll help Serbia more by going abroad. The world is your home. Where you find love is where you'll make your home. Be happy that you have an opportunity to meet new people. Open your heart, because that is the only way your heart can give and receive. It can't possibly be as cold in Norway as people say. The Norwegians surely survive there and prosper because they have warmth in their hearts. G–d led you to a path that leads to them. Love them! Love is the engine of survival, and it's the only open secret your heritage holds."

* * * *

I embraced my mother. I would soon have to leave her. A new door has opened: I would have loved to learn more — but I must leave. This discovery afforded me a new perspective in life. Serbia's borders have expanded, which makes it easier for me to leave.

EPILOGUE

Norway — My New Home

In September 1999, I land in Oslo's Gardermoen Airport. The airport is clean, plain, and unpretentious. I was expecting more of an ostentatious display of wealth and luxury from one of the richest countries in the world.

My trips to Krajina and Kosovo filled me with sadness because of all the tragedies that had struck the Balkans, which have been exhausted by war as well as by a decade of sanctions. I'm now trying to escape the horrible flashbacks that still haunt me.

From Oslo, I take a flight in a small plane to an island in southwest Norway where I had been offered a job. I'm finally in Kristiansund.

My new Hospital Director is supposed to meet me at the airport, but I don't know how I'm going to recognize him. I was advised that he was a middle-aged, blue-eyed gentleman who would be wearing a navy blue marine blazer with gold buttons, and that he has an orange-brown beard. How is this description supposed to help me? That's how I imagine all Norwegian men look. My Norwegian Hospital Director appears in the middle of a group hurriedly exiting the small waiting room at the airport. He looks just as if he's emerging from a prophecy. He's a middle-aged, blond man with a beard who's wearing a dark blue jacket with gold buttons. Instead of saying hello, my whole face lights up with a smile. I relax, as if I'm meeting a close friend. This is a good start.

Awaiting me twenty kilometers down the road is a town of 17,000 inhabitants which has been described as "the cleanest town in all of Norway." It deserves that title, and for good reason. It is immaculate and charming. It imparts an atmosphere of privacy — of generosity, warmth, and peace. September here is usually dark and rainy, but this September the weather is as fine as it is in Belgrade, where September is the loveliest month of the year. This happy coincidence encourages me, so I take it as an auspicious sign.

* * * *

It was already mid-winter when I returned to Kristiansund with my children. The airport was frozen, and a powerful, icy wind was sweeping up everything in its path, including my hat, which I was wearing with great dignity until I stepped off the plane. It tumbled farther and farther away over the icy tarmac, as if it were saying good-bye, and then it vanished irretrievably into the darkness. We waited in vain for our luggage. When the conveyor belt at baggage claims finally stopped without producing our luggage, we got worried. What were we going to do without our things? We soon learned that airport staff in Oslo had mistakenly sent our bags to anosther town in Norway that had a similar name: Kristiansand. I stood there with my two children bereft of our personal belongings in a cold country that was as beautiful and warm as when I had first visited. That's what happens to all our first impressions when they collide with reality: they often don't last much longer than our dreams.

In my pocket, I had a letter Marko had given me. He asked me not to open it until I got to Norway. In the envelope was a gold chain with a pendant from his brigade in Glina, where we had met. Officers don't easily part with their decorations. This present made me happy and sad at once. The past was behind me, but I still have to find the right place for it in my thoughts.

Now all I have is a future.